50 Bread Baking Recipes

Easy Bread Recipes with Minimal Ingredients and Step-by-Step Directions on How to Create Bread!

Table of Contents

INTRODUCTION

This book has a collection of Easy Bread recipes with minimal ingredients and step-by-step directions on how to create bread! This book contains the best handmade bread recipes for both beginners and experienced bakers.

Homemade bread is one of the people's favorite foods of all time. There really is nothing quite like a warm slice of fresh bread served with a thick pat of butter on top. This Bread making recipe book is perfect. It's simple to follow, takes about two hours to make, and yields multiple loaves of wonderful bread.

Basic Steps for most bread recipes

If you've never made bread before, here is the basic formula for making your own at home.

STEP 1: ASSEMBLE BREAD INGREDIENTS

Warm water, granulated sugar, instant OR active dry yeast, salt, vegetable or canola oil, and flour are all required ingredients. That's it!

STEP 2: DISSOLVE THE YEAST AND ACTIVATE IT BY PROOFING

This is a quick and easy procedure that takes about five minutes to complete. You can see what yeast looks like after it has been proofed in the image below. If you use too hot water, yeast can be killed, so aim for slightly warmer than lukewarm, or around 105°F. In a mixing bowl, combine warm water, yeast, and one tablespoon of granulated sugar. After a short stir, set it aside for five minutes. You'll begin to see the yeast puff up until it covers the entire surface of the water.

STEP 3: ADD REMAINING INGREDIENTS AND MIX

Add the remaining sugar, oil, salt, and flour (you can use all-purpose flour OR bread flour!) beat with an electric mixer for about two minutes, or until well blended. It is possible to mix by hand, but it will take longer.

STEP 4: KNEAD THE BREAD

"Wait!" you might scream. "It's already mixed!" Ha! Not so quickly! Kneading bread dough is essential for achieving a great texture in the bread. Kneading dough causes gluten to develop, allowing it to rise higher, be lighter, and fluffier. Kneading can be done by hand or with a mixer. Knead for seven minutes using the dough hook on your machine. If you knead by hand, you'll want to knead for ten-eleven minutes, depending on how consistent you are.

STEP 5: FIRST RISE

Cover your lovely smooth, elastic bread dough with plastic wrap or a clean towel in an oiled dish. Plastic wrap works better since it keeps heated air inside, requiring a shorter first rise for the dough. Make sure to grease the side of the plastic wrap that will come into contact with the dough!

Your bread will take longer to rise if your house is cool. When my house is cooler than usual in the winter, we prefer to turn on the oven for two-three minutes, then turn it off and leave the dough bowl in there to rise. The heat is trapped in the oven for a long time, making it ideal for rising dough.

STEP 6: PUNCH DOUGH AND SHAPE IT

Punching the dough down releases any air pockets that have formed, resulting in a more consistent rise and texture for your Bread. Form your dough into an oblong ball by shaping it gently into a ball and rolling it two or three times on the table. After that, please put it in a greased bread pan.

STEP 7: SECOND RISE

Turn on the oven immediately before punching down the dough, then turn it off once the dough is in the oven for the second rise. It's only on for a minute or two, which is perfectly OK! The second rise, which takes around thirty minutes, will help shape your loaf of bread.

After that, all you need is to bake the prepared bread and then enjoy it.

So, What are you waiting for? Let's get into the universe of delicious bread-making recipes!

SOURDOUGH BREAD

Preparation: 10 Minutes

Cook: 25 Minutes

Servings: 8

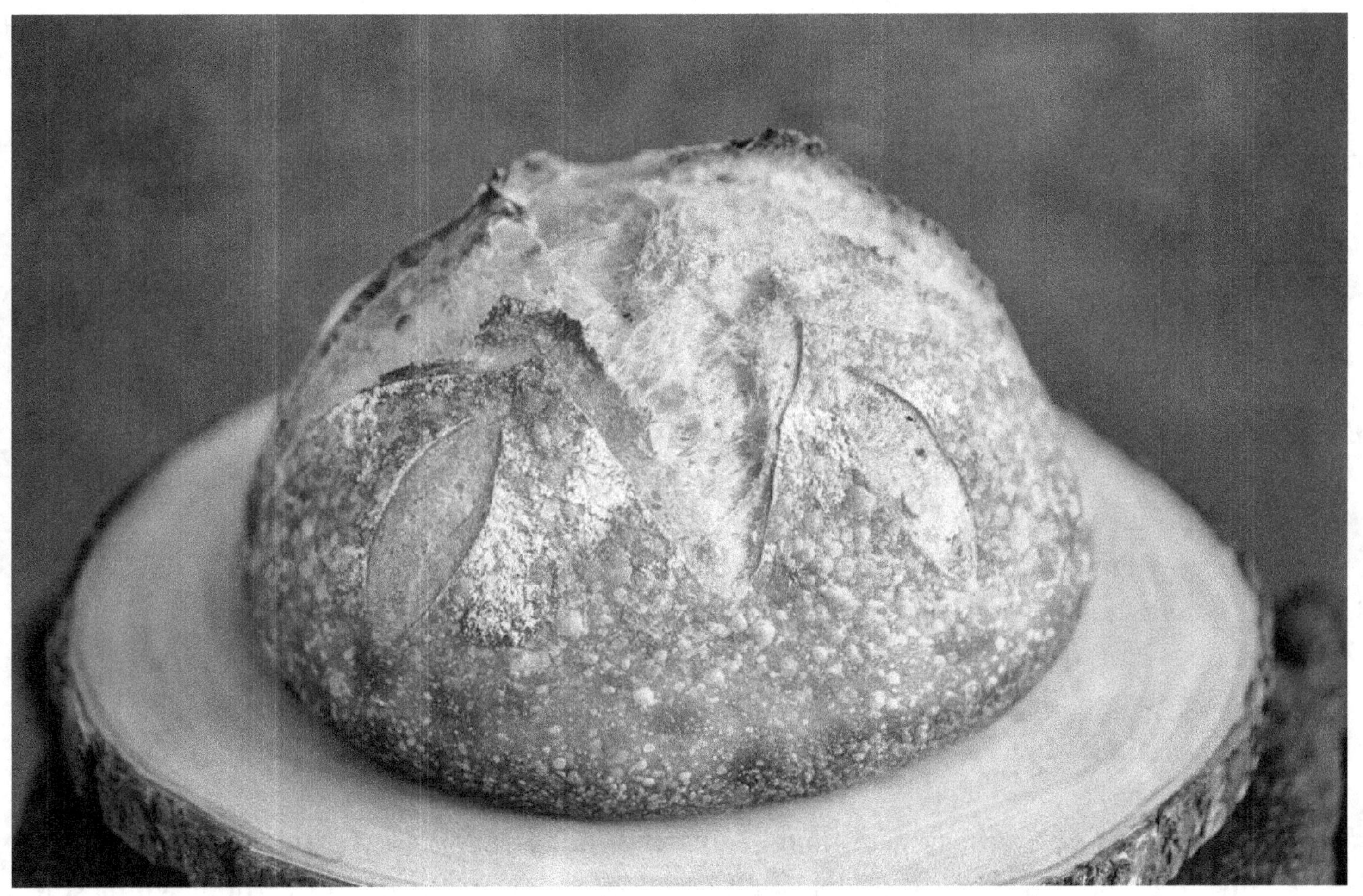

Making your sourdough bread takes a little time, but the actual work is minimal—and the results are fantastic

Nutrition

Calories: 205 | Protein: 6.9g | Cholesterol: 0.1mg | Sodium: 404.8mg

Carbohydrates: 41.2g | Fat: 0.9g

Ingredients

- 250 grams water
- 394 grams bread flour
- Rice flour for bread form
- 100 grams sourdough starter
- 8 grams kosher salt
- 1 10-inch banneton

Instructions

1. Fill a bowl halfway with the starter. Combine the water, salt, and bread flour in a mixing bowl. Mix until all of the ingredients are thoroughly combined into a very sticky dough. Cover with aluminum foil and set aside for four hours at 70-75°F
2. Fold the dough three or four times over on itself with damp hands. Cover with foil and let aside for another two hours to ferment.
3. Dust a bread mold lightly with rice flour.
4. Scrape the dough onto a floured work surface. Make a smooth, unbroken ball with just enough flour on the surface to keep it from sticking together. Place the smooth side down in the banneton. To preserve the round ball shape, pinch together the rougher corners of the surface toward the center to smooth them down.
5. To slow the fermentation process, cover and refrigerate for twelve hours.
6. Remove the loaf from the refrigerator and place it in a warm place to rise for three to five hours, or until the dough springs back slowly and retains a little indentation when lightly poked with a finger.
7. Preheat the oven to 450 degrees Fahrenheit. Using parchment paper, line a rimmed baking sheet.
8. Dust the dough's surface with flour. Transfer dough to parchment paper by gently inverting the banneton over the baking sheet. Brush away any extra rice flour with a soft brush. With a sharp knife, score the top of the dough approximately 1/8-inch deep to form a shallow slit running across the middle. Using a light mist, softly spray the entire surface.
9. Bake for twenty-five to thirty minutes in the center of a preheated oven until beautifully browned. Place on a cooling rack to cool completely.

STRAWBERRY BREAD

Preparation: 30 Minutes

Cook: 45 Minutes

Servings: 24

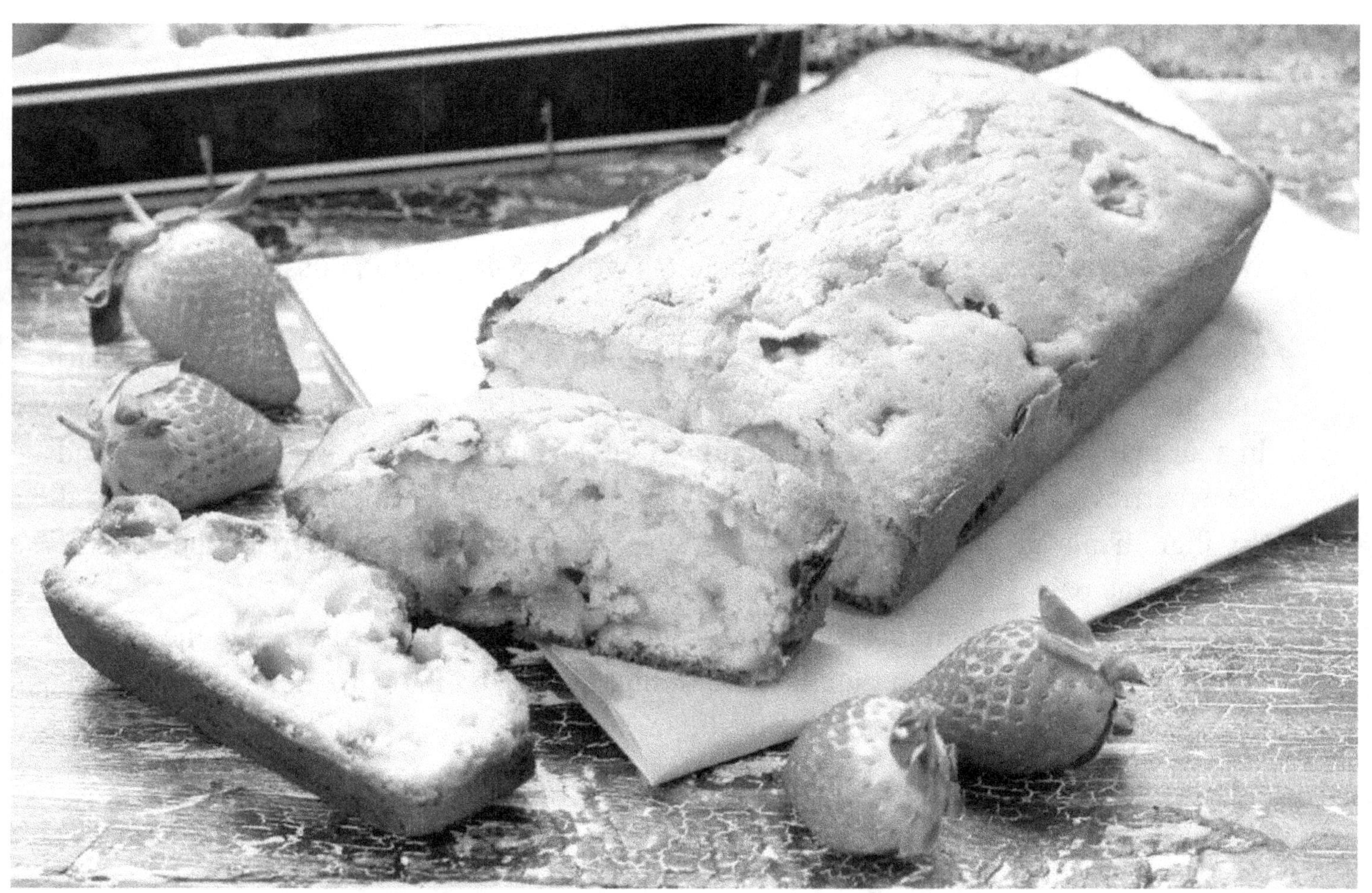

This dish is delicious hot or cold, as a breakfast or dessert. This is a family favorite!

Nutrition

Calories: 281 | Protein: 3.3g | Cholesterol: 31mg | Sodium: 161.5mg

Carbohydrates: 31.2g | Fat: 16.6g

Ingredients

- 4 eggs, beaten
- 2 cups white sugar
- 2 cups fresh strawberries
- 1 ¼ cups chopped pecans
- 3 ⅛ cups all-purpose flour
- 1 ¼ cups vegetable oil
- 1 tablespoon ground cinnamon
- 1 teaspoon baking soda
- 1 teaspoon salt

Instructions

1. Preheat the oven to 350 degrees Fahrenheit. Two 9 x 5-inch loaf pans ought to be butter and flour.
2. Strawberries must be sliced and placed in a medium-sized dish. Set aside while preparing the batter with a light dusting of sugar.
3. In a large mixing bowl, whisk together the flour, sugar, cinnamon, salt, and baking soda. Strawberries will be blended with oil and eggs. Blend in the strawberry mixture until the dry ingredients are barely moistened. Add the pecans and mix well. Divide the batter between the pans.
4. Bake forty-five to fifty minutes in a preheated oven until a tester inserted in the center comes out clean. Allow ten minutes for cooling in pans on the wire rack. Remove loaves from pans and set aside to cool before slicing.

WHOLE WHEAT BEER BREAD

Preparation: 10 Minutes

Cook: 50 Minutes

Servings: 12

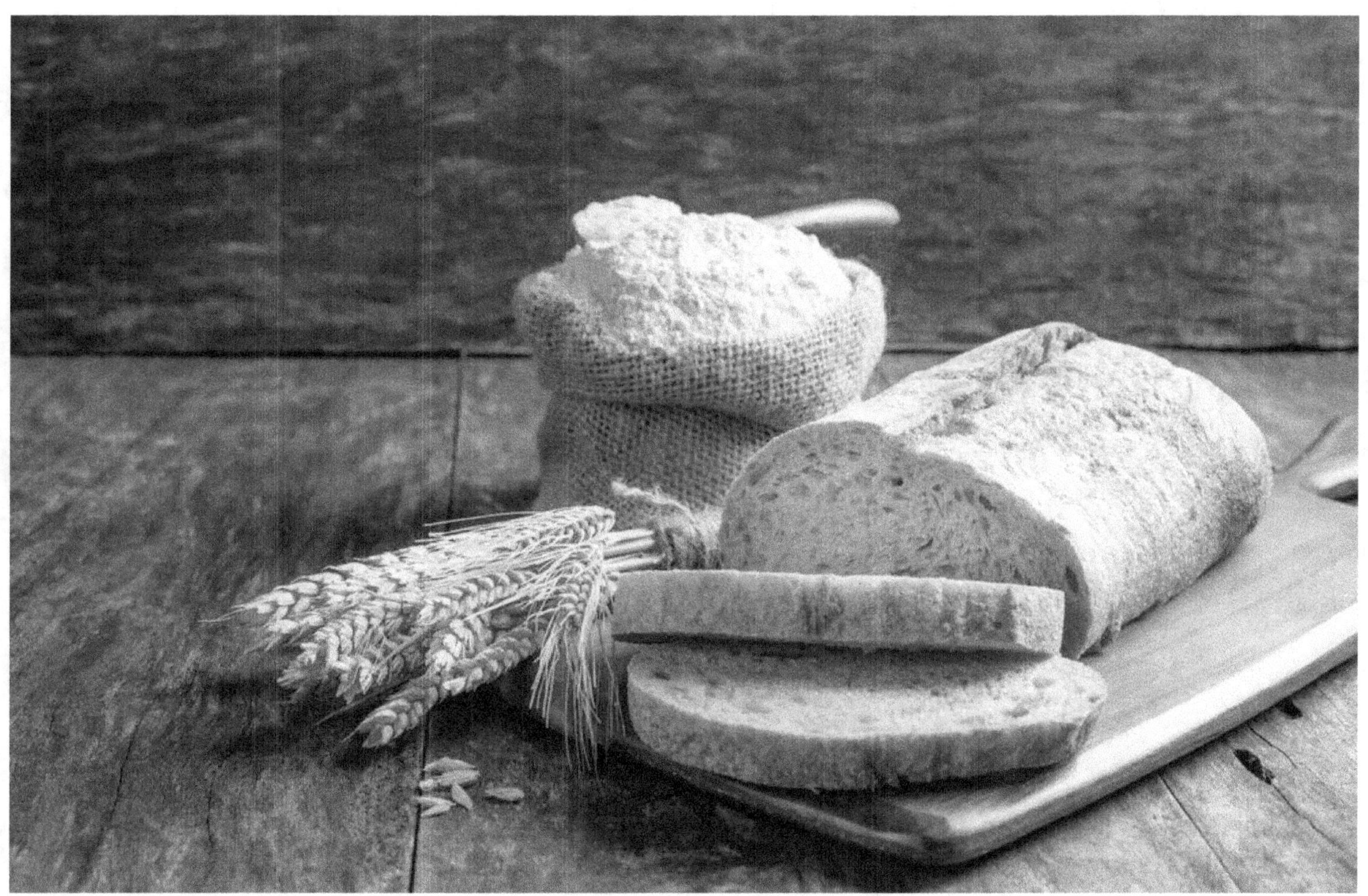

Chili and soups go well together. It makes great toast. Depending on the type of beer used, the flavor of the bread will alter. The top of the loaf seems textured.

Nutrition

Calorics: 144 | Protcin: 3.8g | Fat: 0.4g | Sodium: 429.5mg | Carbohydrates: 30.2g

Ingredients

- ⅓ cup packed brown sugar
- 1 ½ cups whole wheat flour
- 1 ½ cups all-purpose flour
- 4 ½ teaspoons baking powder
- 1 ½ teaspoons salt
- 1 can or bottle of beer

Instructions

1. Preheat the oven to 350 degrees Fahrenheit. Grease a 9x5-inch loaf pan lightly.
2. Combine all-purpose flour, whole wheat flour, baking powder, salt, and brown sugar in a large mixing basin. Pour in the beer and whisk until a firm batter forms. You may have to stir the dough with your hands. Scrape dough into a loaf pan that has been prepared.
3. Bake for fifty to sixty minutes in a preheated oven or until a toothpick inserted in the center of the loaf comes out clean.

GARLIC NAAN

Preparation: 25 Minutes

Cook: 20 Minutes

Servings: 6

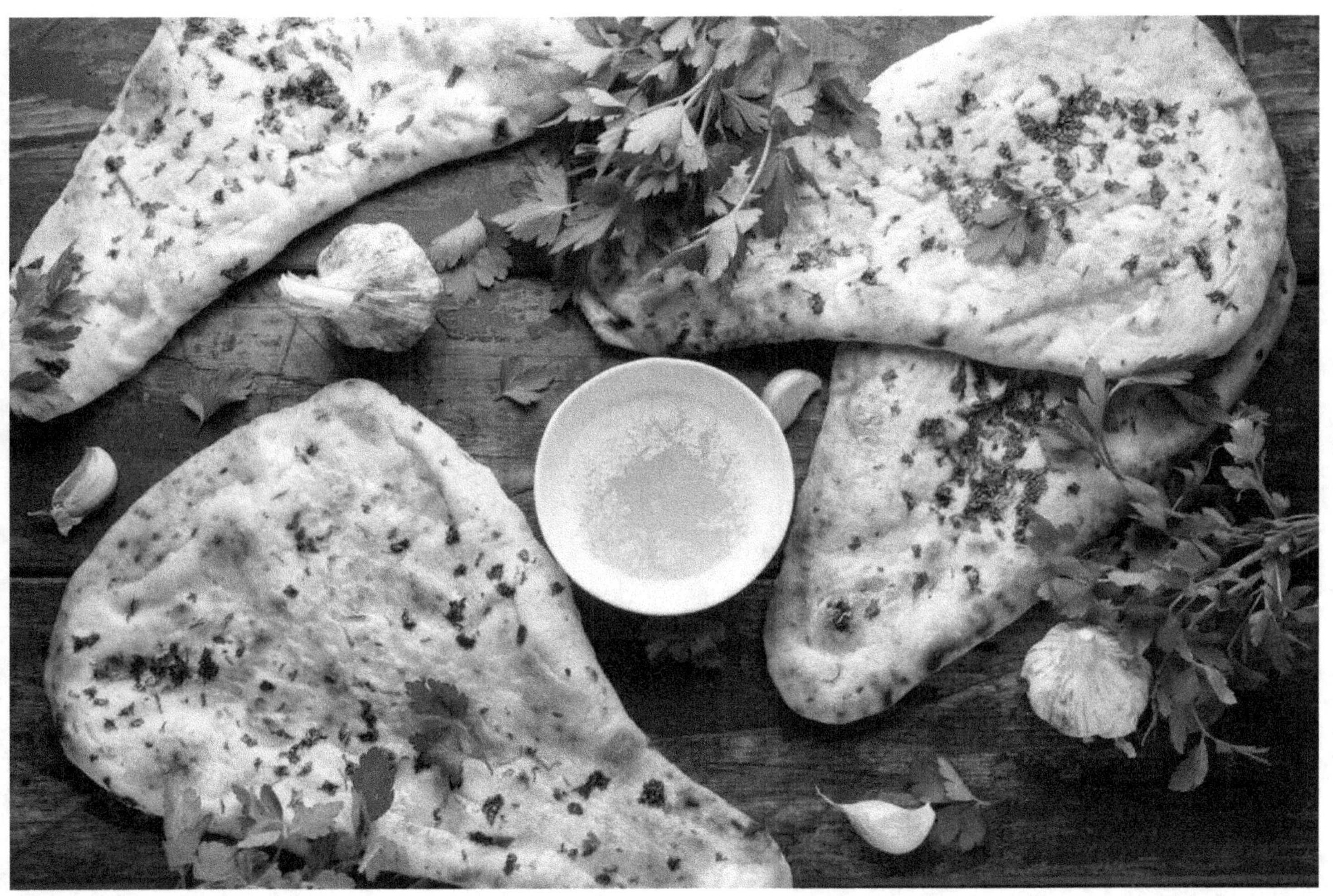

Though restaurant naan is often cooked in the high heat of a tandoor oven, you can make this variation at home in a hot cast iron pan. The naan will produce blistering bubbles with a gorgeous golden-black char when cooked at the correct temperature. Soak it in excessive amounts of curry to reward yourself for a job well done.

Nutrition

Calories: 227 | Protein: 6g | Cholesterol: 20.9mg | Sodium: 384.7mg

Carbohydrates: 31.3g | Fat: 8.6g

Ingredients

- 1 (.25 ounce) package active dry yeast
- 1 teaspoon white sugar
- ½ cup warm water

<u>For the Garlic Butter</u>

- 2 cups bread flour, or more as needed
- ¼ cup plain yogurt
- ¼ cup butter
- ¼ cup chopped cilantro (Optional)
- 2 cloves garlic, minced
- 1 teaspoon kosher salt

Instructions

1. In a mixing bowl, combine the water, sugar, and yeast. Allow approximately fifteen minutes for the yeast to soften and make a creamy foam.
2. Meanwhile, melt the butter in a pan over medium heat until it sizzles. Mix in the garlic right away. Remove the garlic butter from the heat and set it aside until needed.
3. Toss the yeast mixture with the yogurt, bread flour, salt, and 1 tablespoon of garlic butter. Stir until a shaggy dough forms using a wooden spoon. Knead the dough by hand until it pulls away from the bowl's sides, adding more water or flour as necessary. Three to four minutes later, turn the dough out onto the counter and continue kneading it into a smooth ball. In a large mixing bowl, place the dough. Drizzle a couple of additional drizzles of garlic butter on top. Cover and let rise for about two hours, or until doubled in volume.
4. Turn out the dough onto the counter after punching it down. Cut into 6 pieces after forming a rough rectangle. Each piece should be rolled into a ball and lightly dusted with flour. Cover with plastic wrap and proof for fifteen to twenty minutes, or until somewhat puffy.
5. Each piece will be rolled into an oval about 1/8 inch thick. Sprinkle some cilantro on top and lightly press it in place.
6. Preheat a cast-iron skillet for about 5 minutes or until it is quite hot. Cook each naan for one to two minutes, or until large bubbles appear. Flip over, carefully push down, and cook for another two to three minutes, or until bubbles on the bottom are scorched. Before serving, brush the naan with additional garlic butter.

BROWN BUTTER PINEAPPLE CORN MUFFINS

Preparation: 10 Minutes

Cook: 25 Minutes

Servings: 12

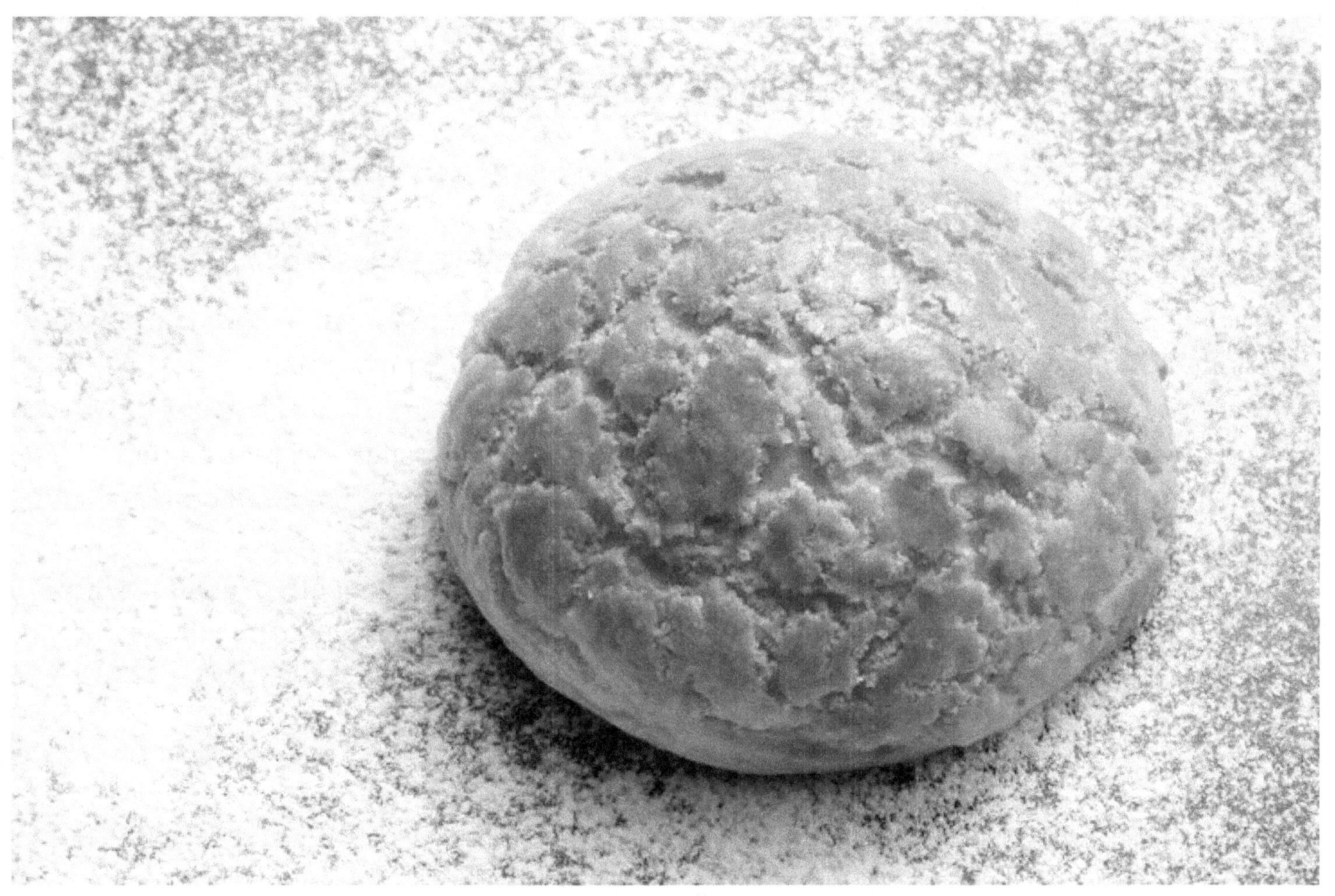

When you're talking about cornbread, you're also talking about a big bowl of chili, and nothing balances that big spoon in one hand like a warm corn muffin in the other.

Nutrition

Calories: 195 | Protein: 4g | Cholesterol: 52.2mg | Sodium: 185.6mg

Carbohydrates: 24.1g | Fat: 9.2g

Ingredients

- 2 large eggs
- 1 cup all-purpose flour
- ¾ cup chopped dried sweetened pineapple
- 1 cup yellow cornmeal
- ½ teaspoon baking soda
- 1 cup buttermilk
- ½ cup unsalted butter
- ½ teaspoon salt

Instructions

1. Preheat the oven to 375 degrees Fahrenheit. Spray a muffin pan with cooking spray and line it with paper muffin liners.
2. In a big saucepan, melt butter over medium heat until golden brown. Set aside for twenty minutes to steep. Remove the pan from the heat and add the pineapple.
3. Combine flour, cornmeal, baking soda, and salt in a mixing bowl. Set aside.
4. In a large mixing bowl, whisk together the buttermilk, eggs, and pineapple mixture. Whisk one minute until smooth Whisk the flour mixture into the buttermilk mixture until it is completely mixed
5. Bake until a toothpick inserted in the center of a muffin comes out clean, about twenty-five minutes, after evenly dividing the batter between the prepared muffin cups. Cool for five minutes in the pan before removing to a wire rack to cool fully.

BURGER OR HOT DOG BUNS

Preparation: 20 Minutes

Cook: 10 Minutes

Servings: 12

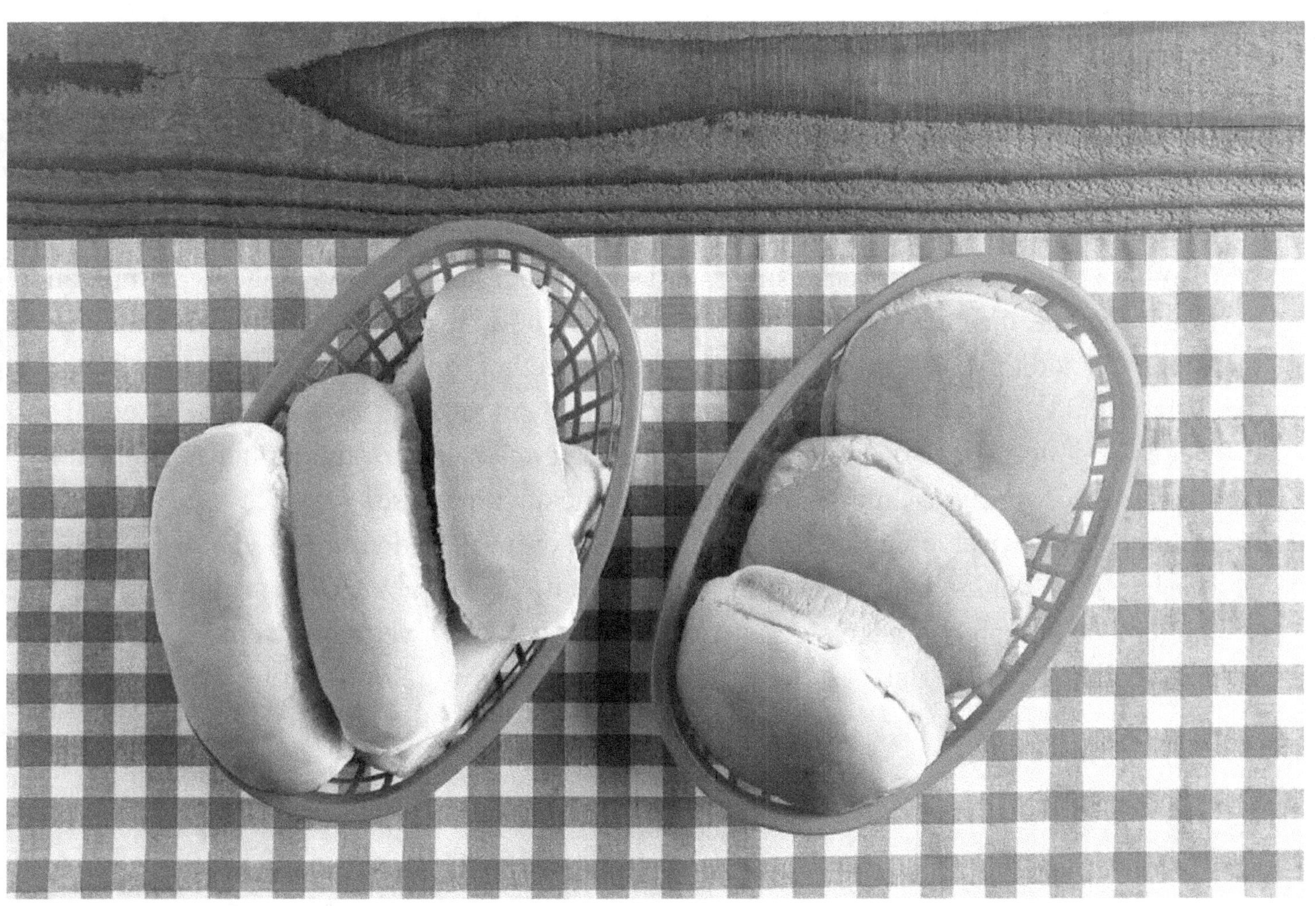

This recipe works well for both hamburger and hot dog buns. They're 'top of the line,' according to my hubby. Soft and pleasant.

Nutrition

Calories: 230 | Protein: 6.3g | Cholesterol: 27.3mg | Sodium: 333.6mg

Carbohydrates: 39.1g | Fat: 5.1g

Ingredients

- 1 egg
- ½ cup water
- 4 ½ cups all-purpose flour
- 2 tablespoons white sugar
- 1 ½ teaspoons salt
- 1 cup milk
- ¼ cup butter
- 1 package instant yeast

Instructions

1. Heat milk, water, and butter in a small pot until very warm, about 120 degrees F.
2. Combine 1 3/4 cup flour, yeast, sugar, and salt in a large mixing bowl. Mix the milk and flour together, then add the egg. 1/2 cup at a time, add the remaining flour, mixing well after each addition. When the dough has come together, turn it out onto a lightly floured surface and knead for about eight minutes, or until smooth and elastic. Make 12 equal pieces of dough. Place on a prepared baking sheet and roll into smooth balls. Slightly flatten. Allow thirty to thirty-five minutes for the dough to rise.
3. Bake for ten to twelve minutes at 400 degrees F, or until golden brown.
4. For Hot Dog Buns: Make a 6x4 inch rectangle out of each piece. Begin rolling up the longer side and pinching the sides and ends to seal. Allow twenty to twenty-five minutes for the dough to rise. Bake as directed above. These buns are quite large.

HOMEMADE FLOUR BREAD

Preparation: 15 Minutes

Cook: 45 Minutes

Servings: 24

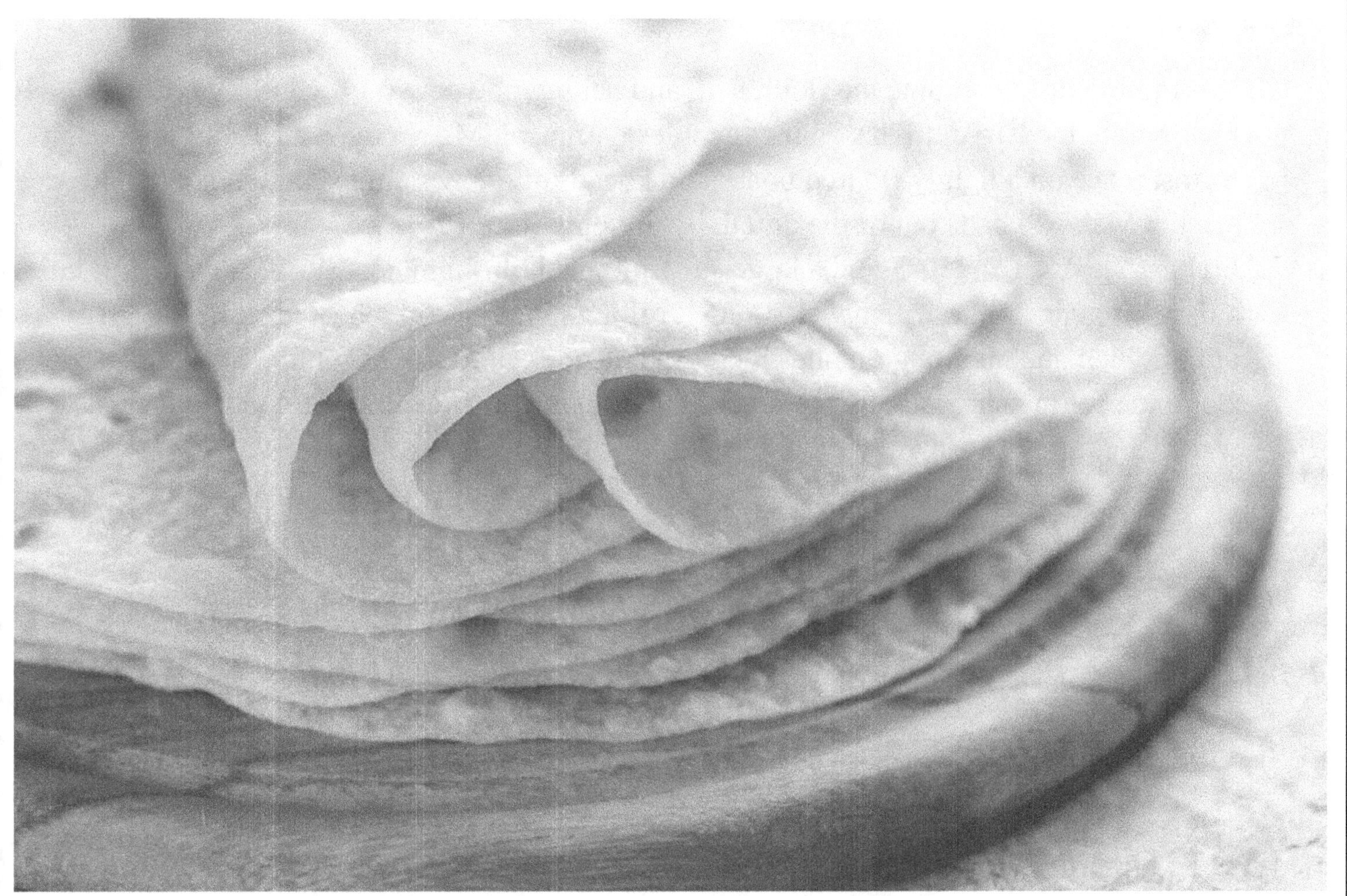

Homemade flour tortillas are far superior to store-bought tortillas. Vegetable oil or shortening can not be used in place of lard

Nutrition

Calories: 86 | Protein: 2.2g | Cholesterol: 1mg | Sodium: 138.4mg

Carbohydrates: 16g | Fat: 1.3g

Ingredients

- 1 ½ cups water
- 2 tablespoons lard
- 4 cups all-purpose flour
- 2 teaspoons baking powder
- 1 teaspoon salt

Instructions

1. In a mixing dish, combine the flour, salt, and baking powder. With your fingertips, incorporate the lard until the flour resembles cornmeal. Mix in the water until the dough forms; place on a lightly floured board and knead for a few minutes until smooth and elastic. Make 24 balls out of the dough by dividing it into 24 equal parts.
2. Preheat the oven to 350°F and a large skillet to medium-high heat. Roll a dough ball into a thin, circular tortilla with a well-floured rolling pin. Place in a heated skillet and fry until golden and bubbling on one side; turn and cook until golden on the other side. Continue rolling and cooking the remaining dough while keeping the cooked tortilla warm in a tortilla warmer.

LEMON BREAD

Preparation: 15 Minutes

Cook: 50 Minutes

Servings: 12

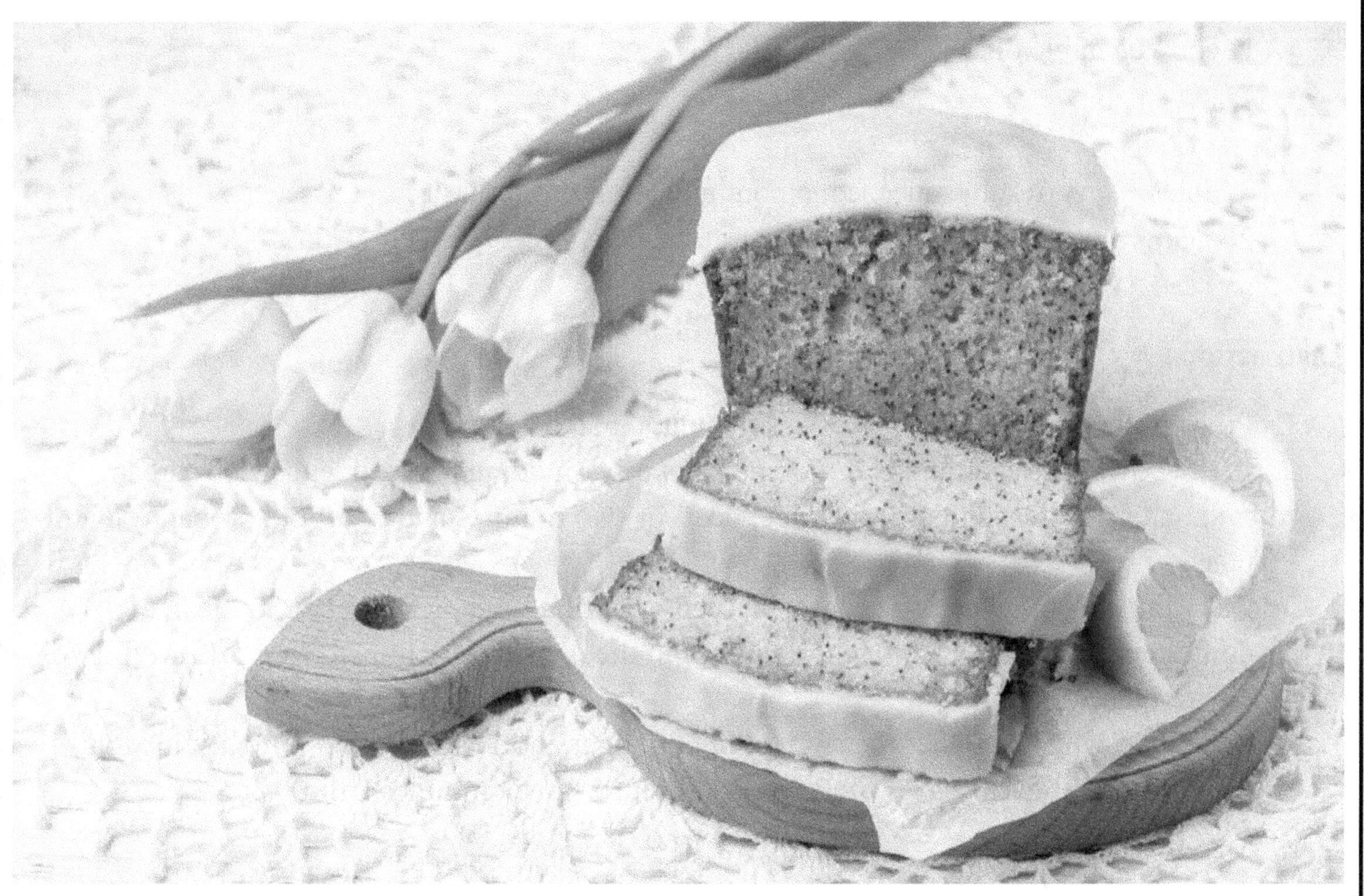

That is the best dish you should make at home. With a cup of freshly prepared coffee, this dish is perfect.

Nutrition

Calories: 477 | Protein: 5g | Cholesterol: 72mg | Sodium: 371.9mg

Carbohydrates: 70.8g | Fat: 20g

Ingredients

<u>Cake</u>

- 4 large eggs
- ½ cup milk
- 6 tablespoons freshly squeezed lemon juice
- package yellow cake mix
- 1 package non-instant lemon pudding mix
- 8 ounces sour cream
- ½ cup vegetable oil

<u>Icing</u>

- 3 tablespoons freshly squeezed lemon juice, or more to taste
- 2 ½ cups confectioners' sugar

Instructions

1. Preheat the oven to 350 degrees Fahrenheit. Grease 2 loaf pans.
2. In the bowl of a stand mixer, combine cake mix, pudding mix, oil, eggs, sour cream, milk, and 6 tablespoons lemon juice; beat for two minutes and pour into prepared loaf pans.
3. Bake for fifty minutes in a preheated oven or until a toothpick inserted in the center comes out clean. Cool for twenty minutes in the pans before transferring to cool fully on a wire rack.
4. In a bowl, whisk together the confectioners' sugar and 3 tablespoons lemon juice until smooth; spoon evenly over the loaves and set for thirty minutes before slicing.

DIANA'S HAWAIIAN BREAD ROLLS

Preparation: 20 Minutes

Cook: 15 Minutes

Servings: 12

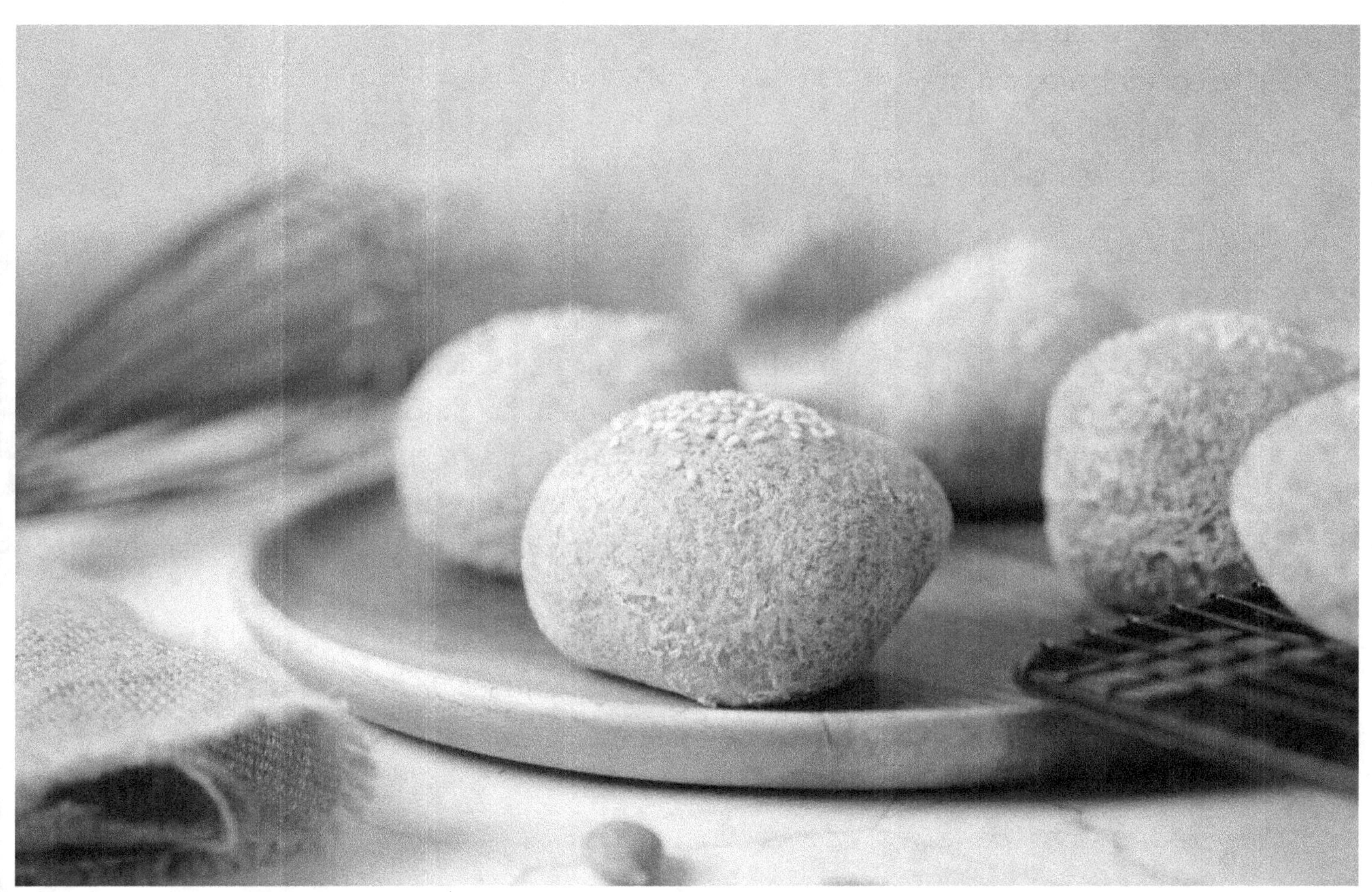

We finally perfected the recipe after years of trying! The greatest dinner rolls are made with this recipe. It's sweet and flavorful. It's a hit with my family and neighbors.

Nutrition

Calories: 64 | Protein: 1.2g | Cholesterol: 15.7mg | Sodium: 208.2mg

Carbohydrates: 8.9g | Fat: 2.6g

Ingredients

- 1 egg
- 4 ½ cups bread flour
- tablespoons white sugar
- 2 tablespoons dry milk powder
- 1 teaspoon salt
- 2 tablespoons butter-flavored shortening 1 ½ cups warm water
- 1 tablespoon molasses
- 1 teaspoon vanilla extract
- 1 teaspoon lemon extract
- 1 tablespoon honey
- 2 teaspoons active dry yeast

Instructions

1. Place the ingredients in the bread machine pan in the manufacturer's recommended order. Press Start after selecting the dough cycle for a 2-pound batch. Because the dough can be a little sticky, you may need to add a little extra bread flour as it comes together.
2. Turn the risen dough out onto a lightly floured board and divide it into twelve equal pieces when the dough cycle is finished. Form the pieces into rounds and lay them on gently oiled baking sheets.
3. Cover the rolls with a moist cloth and let rise for about forty minutes, or until doubled in volume. Preheat the oven to 350 degrees F in the meantime.
4. Bake for fifteen minutes, or until golden brown, in a preheated oven.

SUN-DRIED TOMATO

Preparation: 30 Minutes

Cook: 20 Minutes

Servings: 6

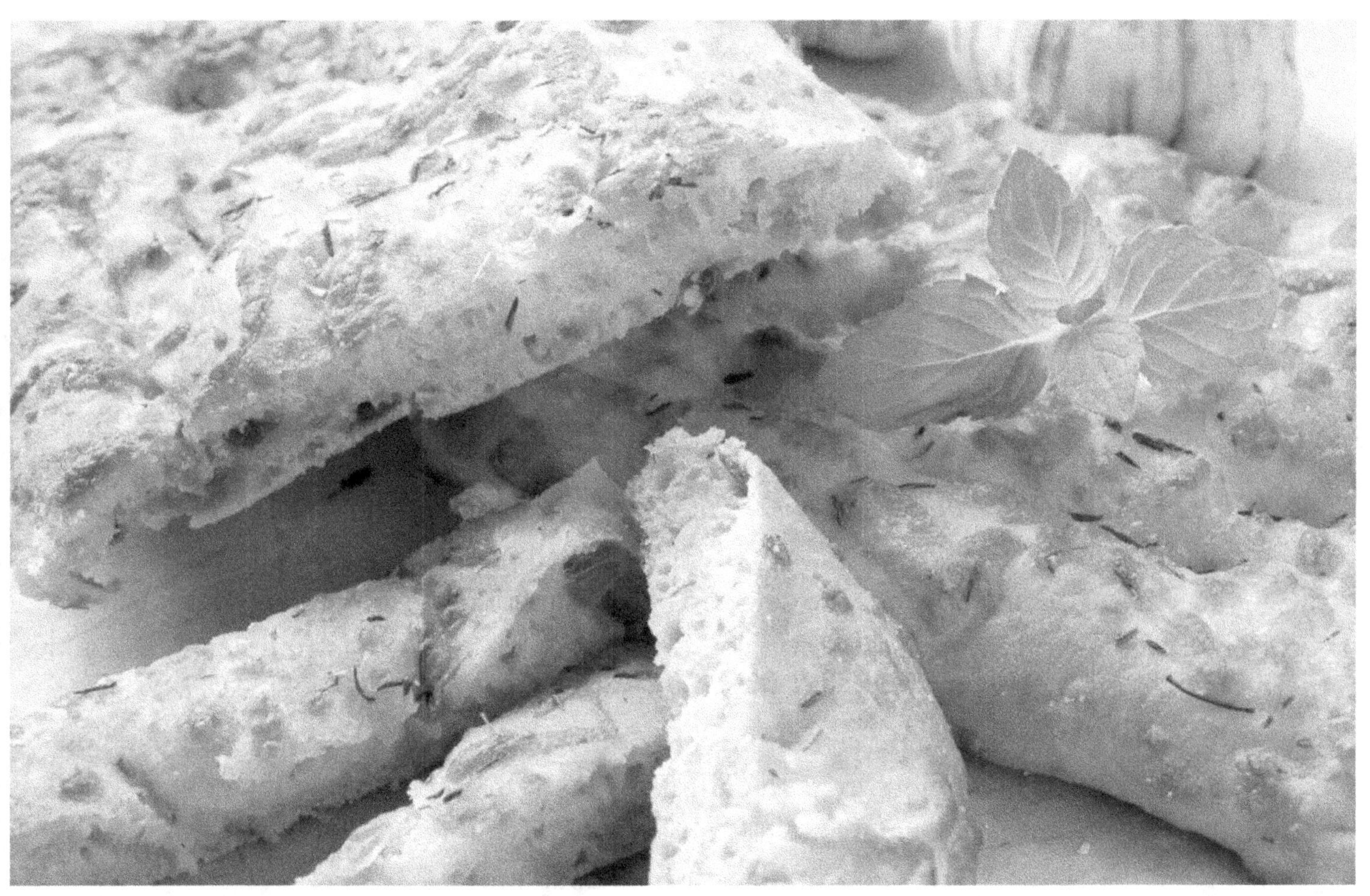

Sun-dried tomatoes, Parmesan, and mozzarella are among the ingredients in this focaccia. This isn't just bread; it's a meal. A cheese-topped cheesy Foccacia.

Nutrition

Calories: 205 | Protein: 6.9g | Cholesterol: 16.7mg | Sodium: 1002.6mg

Carbohydrates: 12.5g | Fat: 14.7g

Ingredients

- 1 cup water
- 2 tablespoons olive oil
- 3 tablespoons margarine
- 2 teaspoons active dry yeast
- 1 cup shredded mozzarella cheese
- 2 teaspoons dried rosemary, crushed
- 3 cups bread flour
- 2 tablespoons dry milk powder
- 3 ½ tablespoons white sugar
- 1 teaspoon salt
- 1 teaspoon garlic salt
- ½ cup chopped sun-dried tomatoes
- 2 tablespoons Parmesan cheese

Instructions

1. In the bread machine, combine water, flour, powdered milk, sugar, salt, butter or margarine, tomatoes, and yeast in the sequence recommended by the manufacturer. Start the machine with the dough cycle selected. The dough will weigh half a pound.
2. Remove the dough from the bread maker once the Dough cycle has completed. Knead by hand for one minute. Place the dough in an oiled bowl and stir it a few times to coat the surface. Allow rising for fifteen minutes in a warm location, covered with a moist cloth.
3. Dust a 10 x 15-inch baking tray with cornmeal. To fit the pan, roll out the dough. With your fingertips, make indentations in the dough. Apply oil to the top surface and cover with a moist cloth. Allow thirty minutes for the dough to rise.
4. Parmesan, rosemary, garlic salt, and mozzarella cheese are sprinkled on top.
5. Bake for fifteen minutes at 400 degrees F, or until well browned. Allow it to cool slightly before cutting into squares to serve.

MICHAEL'S FOCCACIA BREAD

Preparation: 20 Minutes

Cook: 20 Minutes

Servings: 12

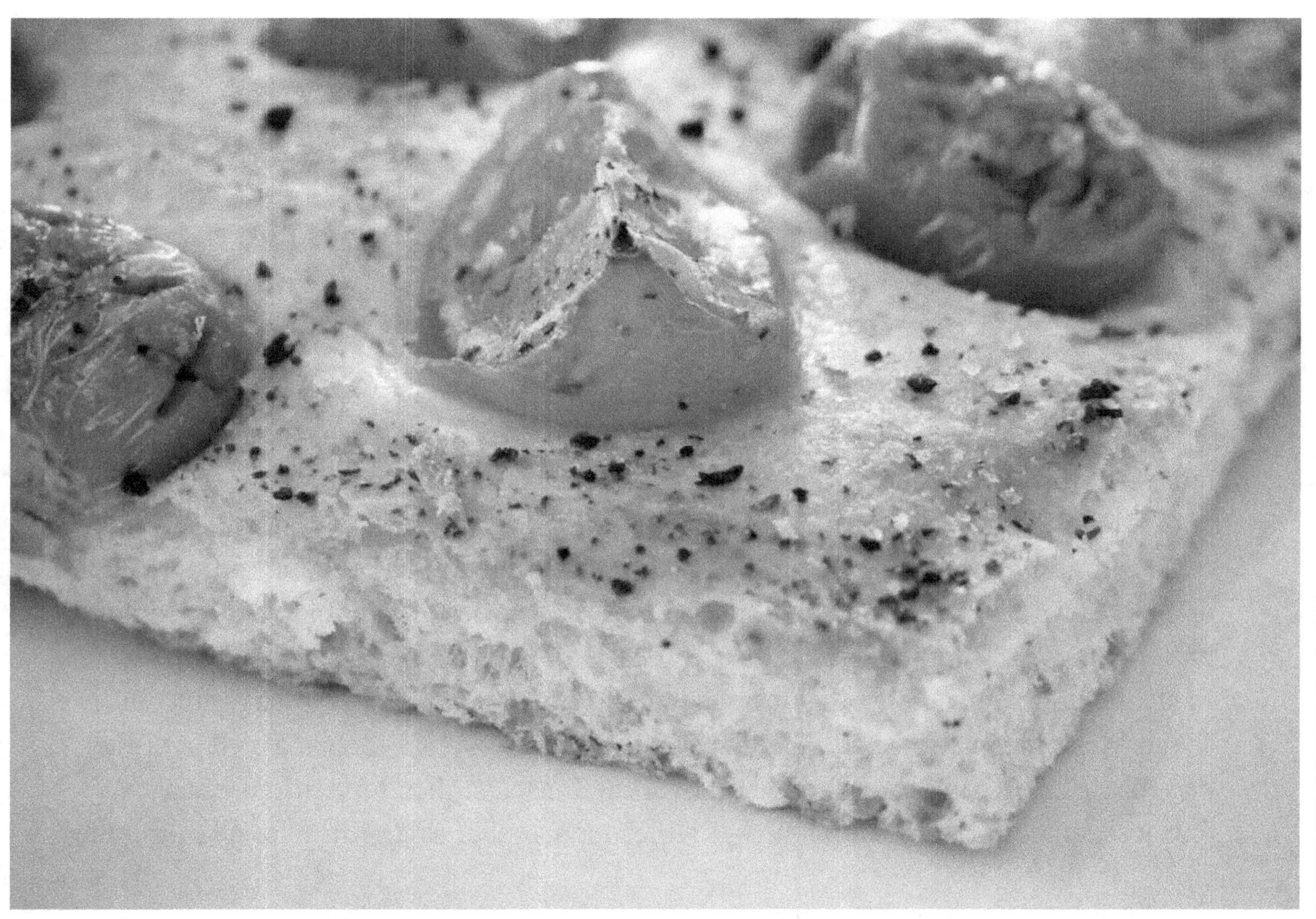

This classic recipe is simple to prepare while keeping authentic and faithful to the original "This may be the quickest yeast bread you've ever made; from start to finish, it just takes one hour. Instead of Parmesan, Romano, or Asiago, cheeses are delicious.

Nutrition

Calories: 249 | Protein: 6.5g | Cholesterol: 1.5mg | Sodium: 987.4mg

Carbohydrates: 42.3g | Fat: 5.6g

Ingredients

- 5 cups all-purpose flour, or as needed
- 3 tablespoons extra-virgin olive oil
- 2 tablespoons fresh chopped rosemary
- ¼ cup freshly grated Parmesan cheese
- 1 tablespoon active dry yeast
- 1 tablespoon honey
- ½ cup diced onion
- 2 cups warm water
- 1 tablespoon kosher salt
- 1 tablespoon extra-virgin olive oil
- 1 tablespoon kosher salt

Instructions

1. In a large mixing dish, dissolve honey in warm water, then sprinkle yeast on top. Allow sitting for five minutes or until the yeast softens and foams. 1 tablespoon salt, 1 tablespoon olive oil, onions, and 5 cups flour will be stirred together until the dough comes together. Knead for five minutes on a well-floured surface until smooth and elastic. Lightly grease a large mixing bowl, then set the dough in it and turn to coat it in oil. Cover with a wet towel and let rise in a warm location for about twenty minutes, or until doubled in volume. Preheat the oven to 415 degrees Fahrenheit.
2. Place the dough on an oiled baking sheet and press it down evenly to cover the entire sheet. Make indentations with the tips of your fingers about 1 inch apart all over the dough. Drizzle 3 tablespoons olive oil over the focaccia, then top with rosemary, Parmesan cheese, and the remaining 1 tablespoon kosher salt. Allow for a ten-minute rise.
3. Bake for twenty minutes, or until golden brown, in a preheated oven.

DECORATED FOCACCIA BREAD

Preparation: 30 Minutes

Cook: 35 Minutes

Servings: 12

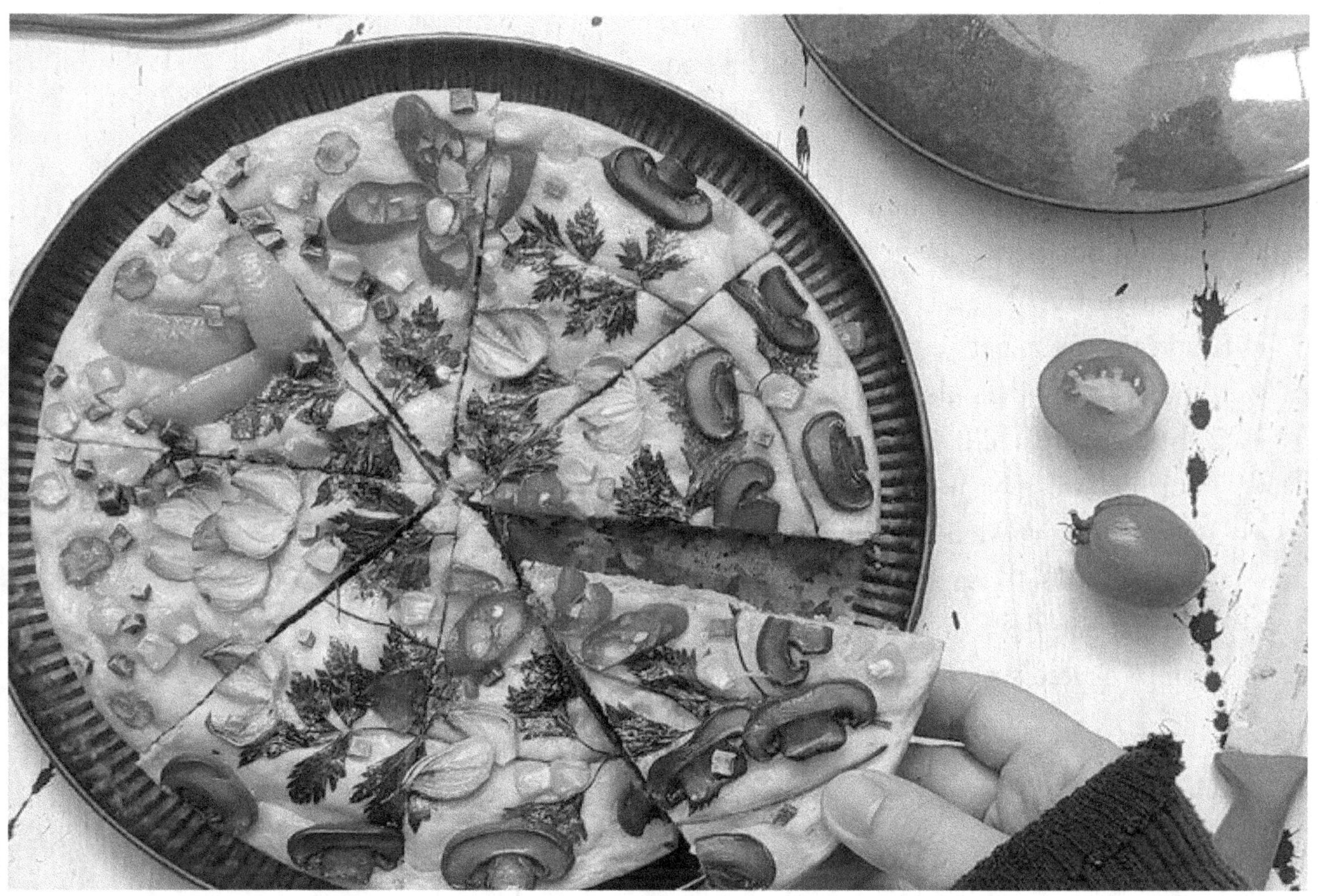

This perfect focaccia is a work of art and a wonderful bite of bread. It's made with typical yeasted dough plus a little milk to help the yeast rise and provide taste. It appears to be a difficult endeavor, yet it comes together quickly. Don't be put off by the prep time; most of the work is done while the dough rises.

Nutrition

Calories: 273 | Protein: 7.1g | Cholesterol: 1.6mg | Sodium: 355.2mg

Carbohydrates: 40.9g | Fat: 9g

Ingredients

<u>Dough</u>

- ¼ cup olive oil
- 1 cup warm water
- 1 cup warm milk
- 4 ½ cups unbleached all-purpose flour, divided
- 1 tablespoon active dry yeast
- 5 each cherry tomatoes, halved
- 4 spears pickled asparagus, drained
- 3 each Kalamata olives, pitted and halved
- 2 teaspoons dried Italian herbs
- 1 ¼ teaspoon kosher salt
- 1 tablespoon olive oil, or as needed
- 1 tablespoon pepitas
- 1 sprig of fresh sage
- 1 sprig of fresh parsley
- 1 tablespoon pine nuts
- 2 sprigs of fresh dill
- 1 sprig of fresh basil
- 3 each jarred roasted red peppers, drained and sliced
- 3 each mini bell peppers, sliced
- 1 tablespoon olive oil, or as desired
- 1 pinch flaked sea salt to taste

Instructions

1. In the bowl of a stand mixer fitted with the paddle attachment, combine 2 cups flour, yeast, dried Italian herbs, and salt. 2 minutes after adding warm water, warm milk, and 1/4 cup oil, beat until thoroughly blended. Mix in the remaining flour, 1/2 cup at a time, until a soft and sticky dough forms, switching to a wooden spoon as needed.
2. Scrape down the sides of the bowl, drizzle 1 tablespoon of oil down the sides, and cover loosely with plastic wrap. Allow rising at room temperature for one hour or until doubled in size.
3. An 11x17-inch baking sheet will be oiled.
4. Place the dough on the baking sheet that has been prepared. To fit the entire sheet, gently spread and flatten the dough. Make light dimples in the dough with your fingers all over the surface. Allow for fifteen minutes of resting time at room temperature, uncovered.

5. Preheat the oven to 450 degrees F and place an oven rack in the lowest third.
6. Press cherry tomatoes, asparagus, red peppers, bell peppers, olives, dill, sage, parsley, basil, pine nuts, and pepitas into the dough. Apply a thin layer of olive oil to the surface and season with salt.
7. Bake for fifteen minutes in a preheated oven. Reduce oven temperature to 350 degrees F and bake for another twenty minutes or until brown and bread springs back when gently touched. Allow it to cool for five minutes in the pan before carefully removing it to a cooling rack. Allow it to cool before serving at room temperature.

EASY ROSEMARY BREAD

Preparation: 30 Minutes

Cook: 10 Minutes

Servings: 6

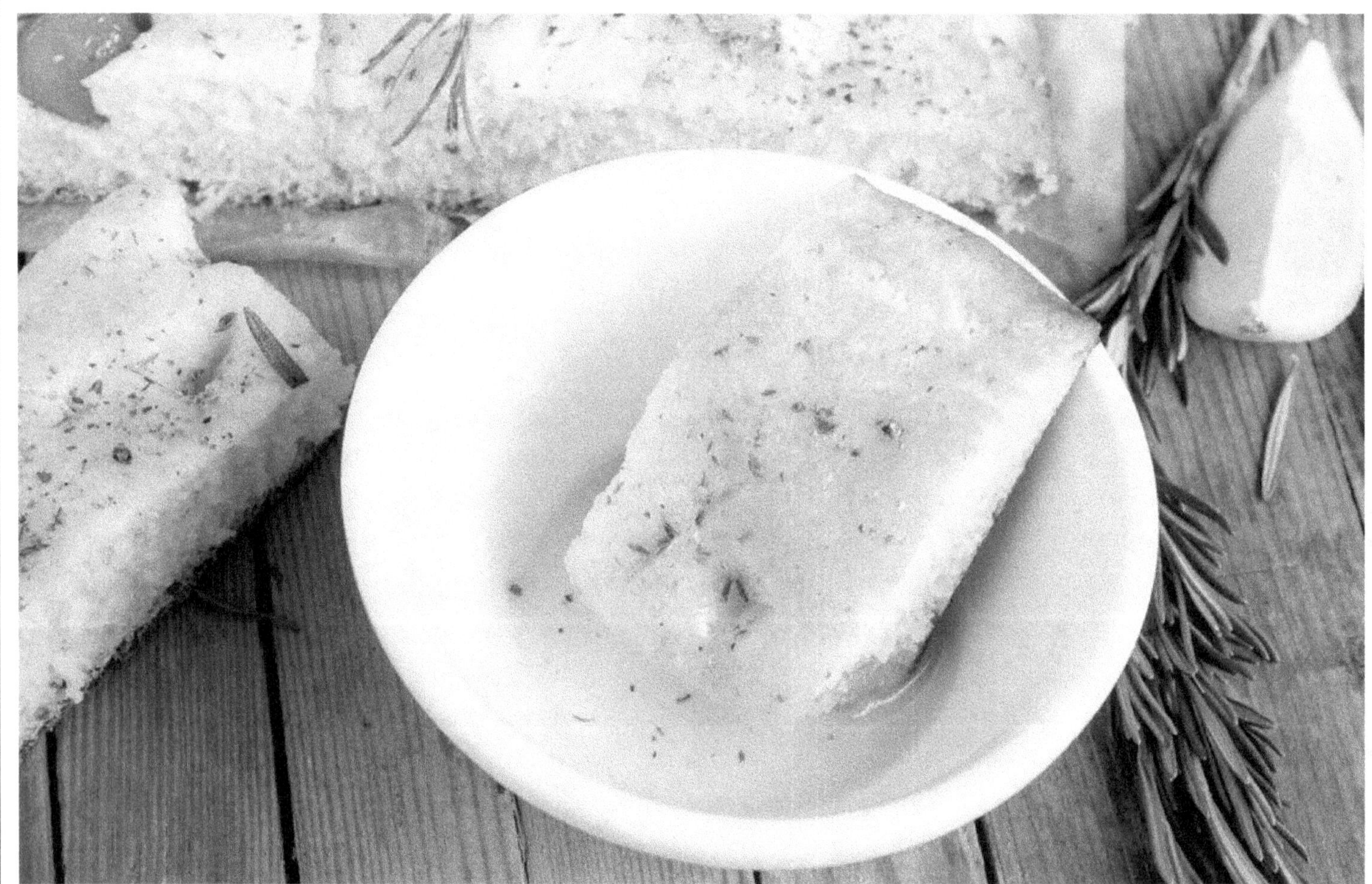

Fresh rosemary and olive oil are used to flavor this simple focaccia bread. So simple, yet so good!

Nutrition

Calories: 299 | Protein: 7.4g | Fat: 7.5g | Sodium: 148.7mg | Carbohydrates: 49.8g

Ingredients

- 2 cups all-purpose flour
- 2 ½ teaspoons active dry yeast
- 1 teaspoon white sugar
- 2 tablespoons olive oil, divided
- 5 tablespoons warm water
- 3 sprigs fresh rosemary, leaves stripped
- ¼ teaspoon salt, or more to taste

Instructions

1. In a large mixing dish, combine 5 tablespoons of warm water, yeast, and sugar. Allow ten minutes for the mixture to become creamy.
2. Toss the yeast mixture with the flour and 1/4 teaspoon salt and whisk well to incorporate. If required, add 1 tablespoon more water at a time until all of the flour has been absorbed. And the mixture has been pulled together into a dough. Turn out onto a lightly floured surface and knead for four to six minutes, or until springy.
3. A large bowl must be lightly oiled. Turn the dough in the bowl to coat it in oil. Cover with a moist towel and set aside in a warm place to rise for thirty minutes or until doubled in volume.
4. Preheat oven to 465 degrees Fahrenheit. Grease a baking sheet lightly.
5. Deflate the dough and place it on a floured surface. Knead the dough briefly, then pat or roll it into a sheet and place it on the baking sheet. Brush the surface with the leftover oil and produce dimples with your fingertips. Toss with rosemary leaves and season with salt and pepper to taste.
6. Bake until crisp, about ten minutes for a light and fluffy or twenty minutes for crunchier and darker on the outside, in a preheated oven.

FOCACCIA DI RECCO

Preparation: 40 Minutes

Cook: 15 Minutes

Servings: 8

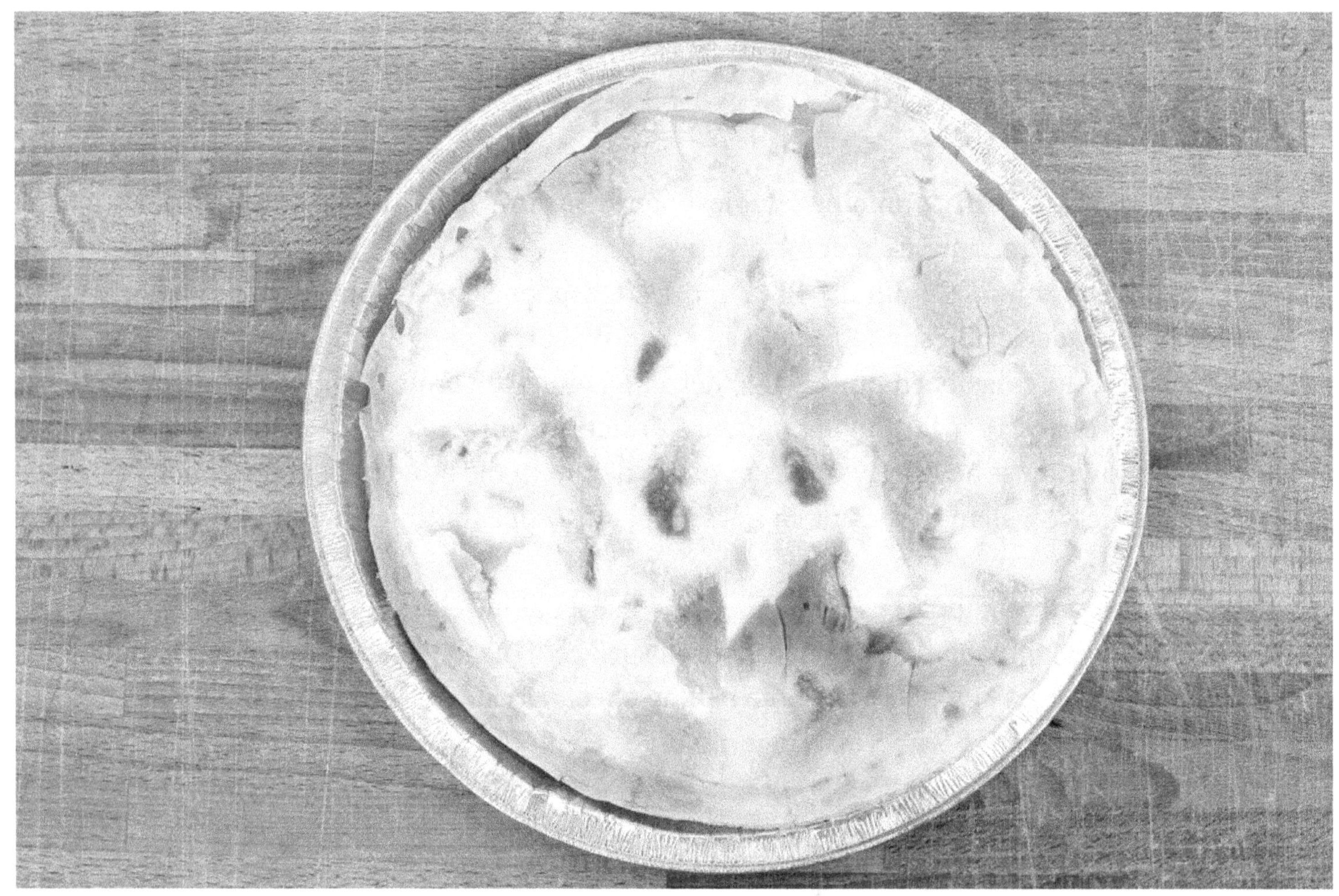

This Ligurian flatbread is tasty and a lot of fun to make. It's delicious on its own, but I prefer it with arugula tossed in a little olive oil.

Nutrition

Calories: 67 | Protein: 4.7g | Carbohydrates: 24.1g | Cholesterol: 7.5mg

Sodium: 326.5mg | Fat: 23.6g

Ingredients

- 12 tablespoons crescenza-stracchino cheese, divided 1 teaspoon extra-virgin olive oil
- 4 teaspoons extra-virgin olive oil, divided
- ¼ teaspoon coarse sea salt, divided
- 1 teaspoon cornmeal
- 1 tablespoon extra-virgin olive oil
- ¾ teaspoon fine salt
- 2 cups all-purpose flour
- ½ cup cold water
- 2 tablespoons cold water
- 1 quarter-sheet baking pan

Instructions

1. Combine flour, both amounts of water, 1 tablespoon olive oil, and 3/4 teaspoon salt in the work bowl of a large stand mixer. Mix dough in a stand mixer fitted with a dough hook on low speed for five to six minutes or until it forms a ball on the dough hook. The dough should be elastic and soft but not sticky.
2. Form a ball with the dough on a work surface. Cover with plastic wrap and set aside for one hour on the counter at room temperature.
3. Lightly grease the quarter-sheet baking pan with 1 teaspoon olive oil; sprinkle with cornmeal. Dust a work surface lightly with flour.
4. Place the oven rack in the middle of the oven. Preheat the oven to 500 degrees Fahrenheit.
5. Cut the dough into quarters after unwrapping it. On a floured work surface, pat each quarter into an approximately rectangle form. 1 piece of dough should be rolled out to about 3/8 inch thick and 6x8 inches in size, keeping the basic rectangular shape. Pick up the dough with well-floured hands and stretch it gently, rotating as you go, until it's almost large enough to cover the prepared sheet pan.
6. Pull and stretch the dough so that it overlaps the pan's edge by approximately 1/2 inch and fastens the dough edges to the sheet pan edges; the dough will be thin and membrane-like.
7. Drop roughly 6 tablespoons of crescenza-stracchino cheese onto the stretched dough and equally distribute the dollops. As before, roll out another piece of dough and stretch it to fit over the first layer of dough and cheese. Stretch, pull, and seal the dough as previously to contain the cheese between the two sheets.
8. Roll a rolling pin over the dough's edges to seal the flatbread edges while also cutting the overlapping edges off. Flatbread will fall into the prepared pan if the overlapping dough

edges are rolled away from the pan. To ensure that the edges of the flatbread are completely sealed, press the flatbread edges flat and roll them slightly if desired. Remove the rolled-off dough edges and toss them out.

9. Pinch a little piece of top dough between your thumb and forefinger and rip a small hole in it; repeat two or three times more to form a few tears in the top layer.

10. Drizzle 2 teaspoons olive oil over flatbread and season with 1/4 teaspoon coarse sea salt.

11. Bake for six to seven minutes in a preheated oven, or until the flatbread has numerous browned, blistered patches on top, the bread has inflated, and the top is crispy. Using the second half of the dough, repeat the instructions to make a second flatbread.

12. Drizzle the remaining 2 teaspoons olive oil and 1/4 teaspoon coarse sea salt over the second flatbread. Bake the second loaf in the same manner as the first. Serve the loaves warm, cut into quarters.

HOMEMADE BAGELS BREAD

Preparation: 30 Minutes

Cook: 20 Minutes

Servings: 6

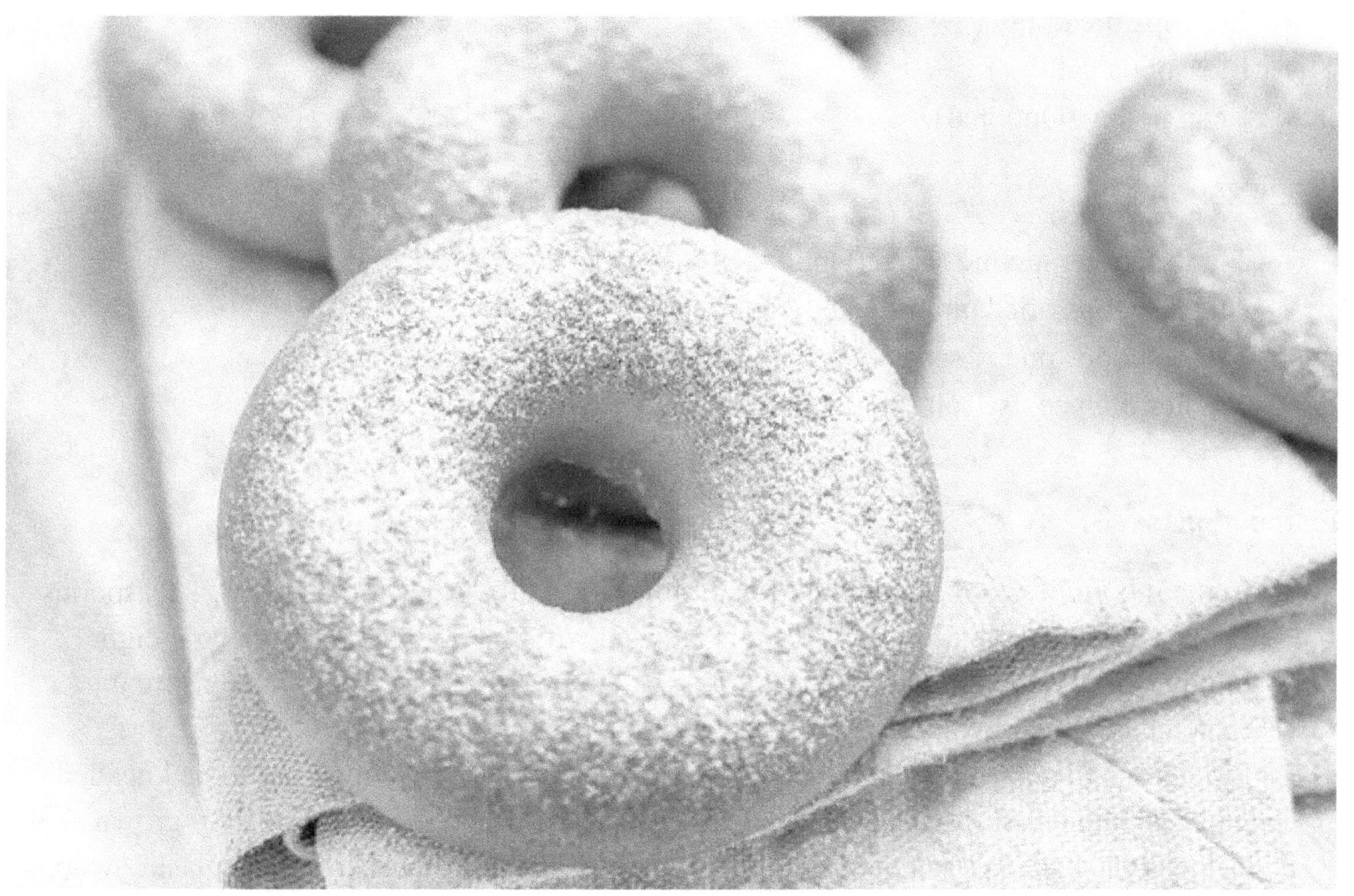

A recipe for the flavor and texture of a traditional bagel.

Nutrition

Calories: 278 | Protcin: 2.1g | Fat: 7.4g | Sodium: 1372.4mg | Carbohydrates: 55.9g

Ingredients

<u>For the Bagels</u>

- 4 quarts water
- 1 ¼ cups water
- 2 tablespoons vegetable oil
- 1 tablespoon instant yeast
- 3 tablespoons white sugar
- 4 ½ cups bread flour
- 1 teaspoon salt
- 1 cup honey (Optional)

<u>Toppings</u>

- 2 tablespoons sesame seeds (Optional)
- 2 tablespoons dried onion flakes (Optional)
- 2 tablespoons poppy seeds (Optional)
- 1 tablespoon coarse salt (Optional)

Instructions

1. In the mixing bowl of a stand mixer, combine 1 1/4 cup water, flour, sugar, 1 teaspoon salt, vegetable oil, and yeast. Mix on low speed with the dough hook for about eight minutes or until well-developed. Cut off a walnut-sized piece of dough to ensure the gluten has fully grown.
2. Flour your fingers and stretch the dough; if it tears easily, the dough has to be kneaded more. A thin translucent "windowpane" should form when the dough is fully grown.
3. Allow the dough to rise for two hours in a lightly oiled dish, covered with plastic wrap and a kitchen towel.
4. Punch down the dough, set it on a lightly floured work surface, and divide it into 6 pieces with a knife or dough scraper (or more, for smaller bagels).
5. Each piece of dough will be rolled into a 6-inch long sausage shape. To make a circle, join the ends together. Repeat with the remaining dough and set aside for fifteen minutes to allow the bagels to rise.
6. Preheat the oven to 475 degrees Fahrenheit. Using parchment paper, line a baking sheet. Next to the baking sheet, place small plates with poppy seeds, sesame seeds, and onion flakes. In a big pot, bring 4 quarts of water to a boil. If desired, drizzle with honey. 3 at a time, boil the bagels until they rise to the top of the saucepan, about 1 minute per side.

With a slotted spoon, remove the bagels and set them on the parchment-lined baking sheet.

7. Dip the tops of the wet bagels in the toppings and lay them on the baking sheet with the seeds facing up. Bake in the preheated oven until the bagels begin to brown, fifteen to twenty minutes. If desired, season with coarse salt.

SHERRILL'S BAGELS

Preparation: 25 Minutes

Cook: 40 Minutes

Servings: 24

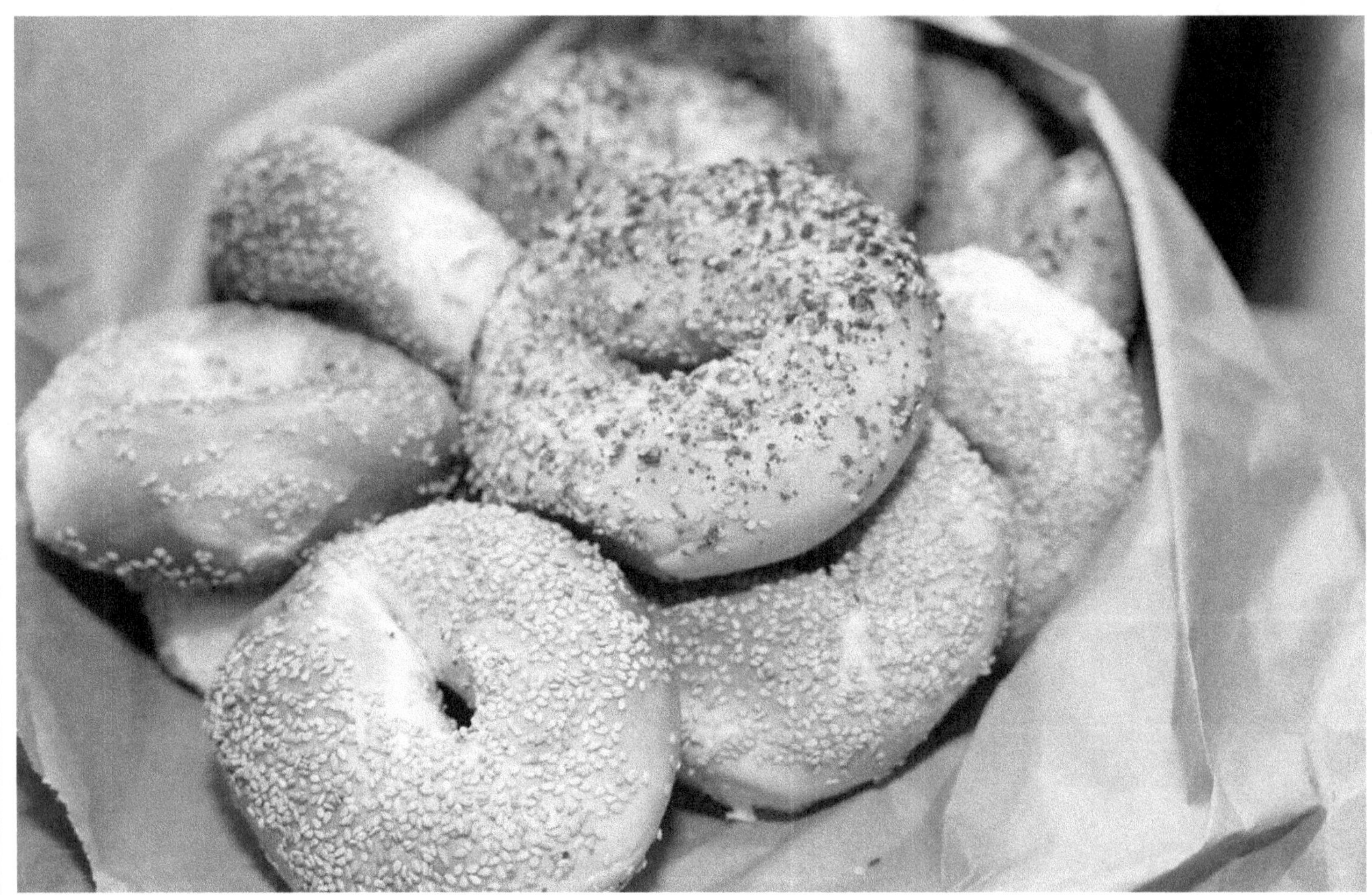

For the past 30 years, every family has had a homegrown tradition of this recipe.

Nutrition

Calories: 180 | Protein: 5g | Fat: 0.5g | Sodium: 292.8mg | Carbohydrates 38g

Ingredients

- 3 cups hot water
- 1 tablespoon salt
- 1 tablespoon dry yeast
- 9 cups all-purpose flour
- ¼ cup white sugar

Instructions

1. In a large mixing bowl, combine flour, boiling water, sugar, yeast, and salt; transfer the dough to a work surface and knead for ten minutes. Allow dough to rise for fifteen minutes in a bowl.
2. Preheat the oven to 375 degrees Fahrenheit. A baking sheet must be greased.
3. Form dough into 24 balls; with a finger, punch a hole in the center of each ball, forming a bagel shape. Allow bagels to rise for twenty minutes on the prepared baking sheet.
4. Bring a large saucepan of water to a boil; cook bagels in batches, about forty-five seconds per side, in the boiling water.
5. Drain the boiled bagels on a clean cloth. Place the bagels back on the baking pan.
6. Bake in the preheated oven until cooked through and lightly browned for thirty to thirty-five minutes.

BREAD MACHINE BAGELS

Preparation: 30 Minutes

Cook: 3 hrs 25 Minutes

Servings: 9

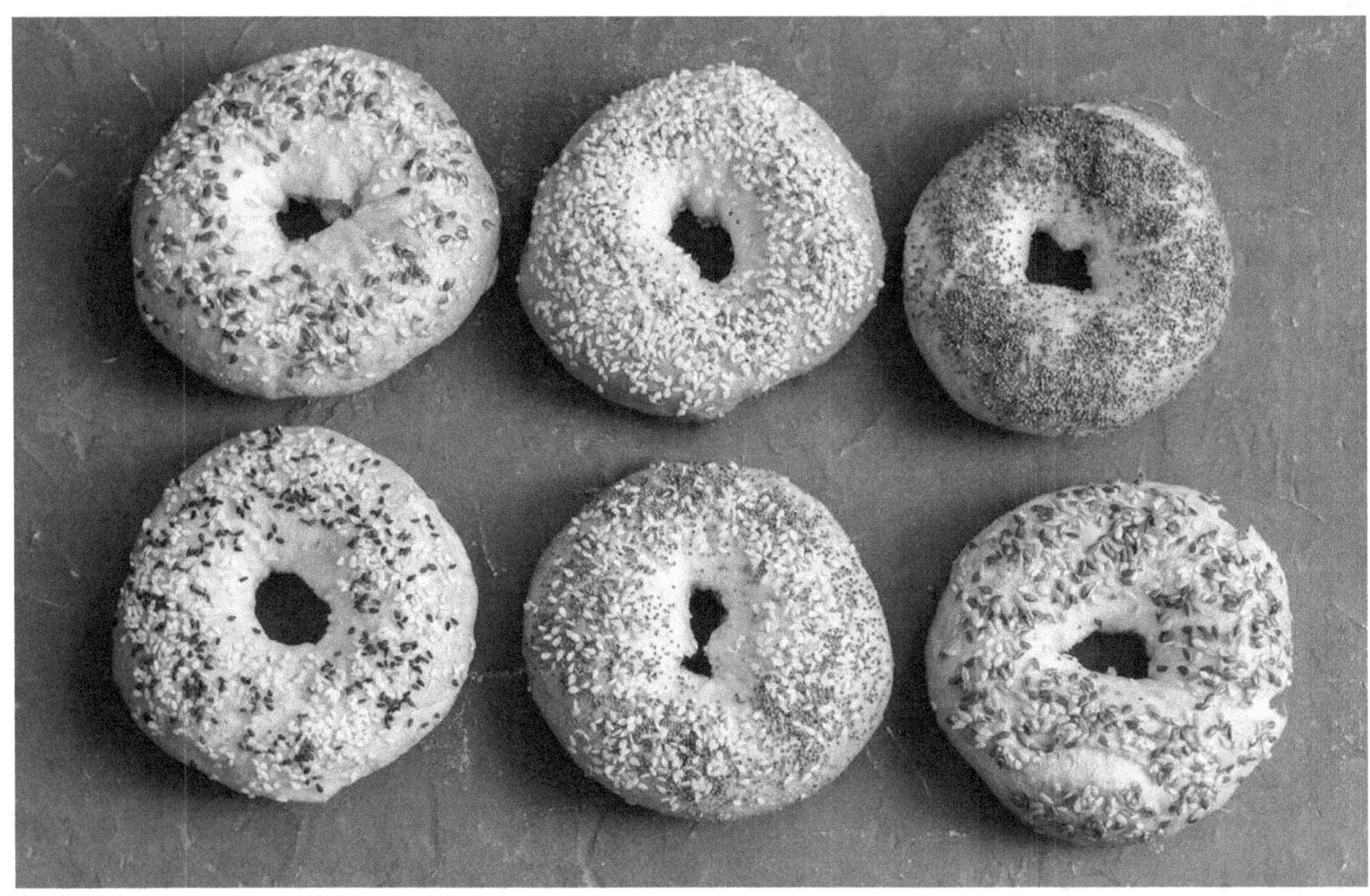

With your bread machine, you can produce quick and easy bagels! You can use any topping you choose, although many people prefer poppy seeds.

Nutrition

Calories: 50 | Protein: 1.4g | Fat: 1.3g | Sodium: 404.4mg | Carbohydrates 8.8g

Ingredients

- 1 egg white
- 3 quarts boiling water
- 3 tablespoons poppy seeds
- 2 ¼ teaspoons active dry yeast
- 2 tablespoons white sugar
- 3 tablespoons white sugar
- 1 cup warm water
- 1 ½ teaspoons salt
- 3 cups bread flour
- 1 tablespoon cornmeal

Instructions

1. In the bread machine pan, add the water, salt, sugar, flour, and yeast in the sequence indicated by the manufacturer. Select the Dough option.
2. Allow dough to rest on a lightly floured surface once the cycle is finished. Meanwhile, bring 3 quarts of water to a boil in a big kettle. Stir in 3 tablespoons of sugar.
3. Make 9 little balls out of the dough by cutting it into 9 equal parts. Make the balls as flat as possible. With your thumb, poke a hole in the middle of each. To enlarge the hole and smooth out the dough around the hole, twist the dough on your finger or thumb. Allow bagels to rest for ten minutes after covering with a clean cloth.
4. Sprinkle an ungreased baking sheet with cornmeal. Transfer the bagels to the boiling water with care. Boil for one minute, turning halfway through. Drain on a clean towel for a few minutes. On a baking sheet, arrange the boiled bagels. Glaze the tops with egg white and top with your favorite toppings.
5. Bake for twenty to twenty-five minutes, until thoroughly browned, in a preheated 375°F oven.

BOILED BAGELS

Preparation: 30 Minutes

Cook: 35 Minutes

Servings: 12

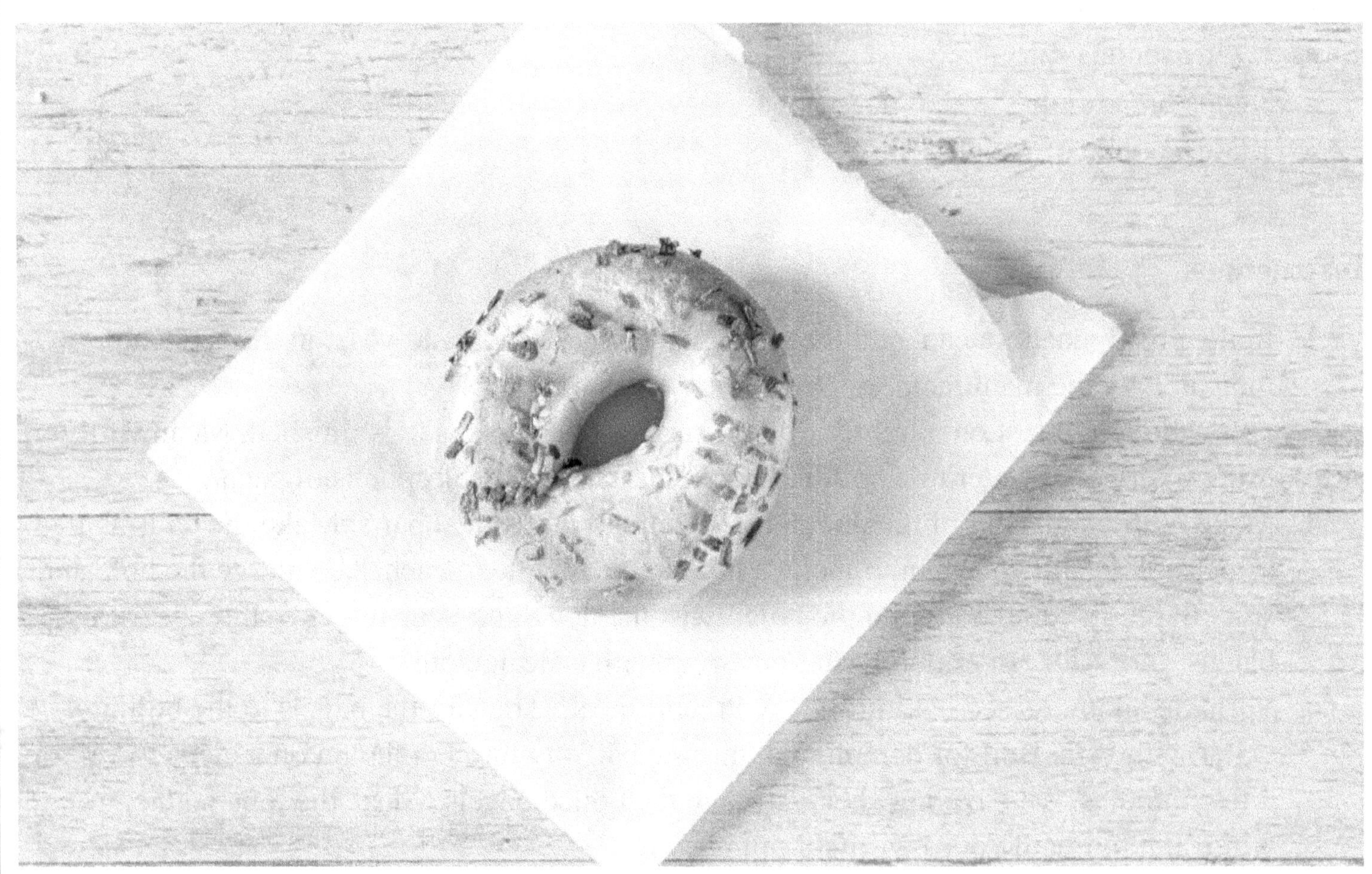

Bagels that have been boiled before baking.

Nutrition

Calories: 181 | Protein: 5g | Fat: 0.5g | Sodium: 583.7mg | Carbohydrates: 38.4g

Ingredients

- 1 tablespoon white sugar
- 1 ½ cups warm water
- 2 packages of active dry yeast
- 3 tablespoons white sugar
- 4 ¼ cups all-purpose flour, or as needed
- 1 tablespoon salt

Instructions

1. Combine 1 1/2 cups flour and yeast in a large mixing basin. Mix the water, 3 tablespoons sugar, and salt in a mixing bowl and stir into the dry ingredients. Scrape the sides of the bowl clean with a mixer for half a minute on low speed. For three minutes, beat at a faster speed. Then, by hand, add enough flour to produce a reasonably stiff dough.
2. Knead the dough on a lightly floured board until it is smooth and elastic. Cover and set aside for fifteen minutes to allow flavors to meld.
3. Cut into 12 pieces and roll into smooth balls. With your finger, poke a hole in the center of the bagel and gently enlarge it while massaging the bagel into a uniform shape. Cover and set aside for twenty minutes to rise.
4. Meanwhile, start heating a gallon of water. Place 1 tablespoon of sugar in it and stir it around. Reduce the heat to a low simmer.
5. Put 4 or 5 bagels in the water when they're done, and cook for 7 minutes, turning once. They should be drained. Bake for thirty to thirty-five minutes at 375 degrees F on a greased baking sheet. Remove from the oven and serve hot or cold.
6. Before boiling, broiling option places elevated bagels on an ungreased baking sheet for a glossier top. Broil them for one to one and half minutes on each side, five inches from the fire. Then, like before, place them in the boiling water. Note: Broiled bagels should not be baked for as long as non-broiled bagels; twenty-five minutes should be enough.

SAN FRANCISCO STYLE BAGELS

Preparation: 30 Minutes

Cook: 30 Minutes

Servings: 8

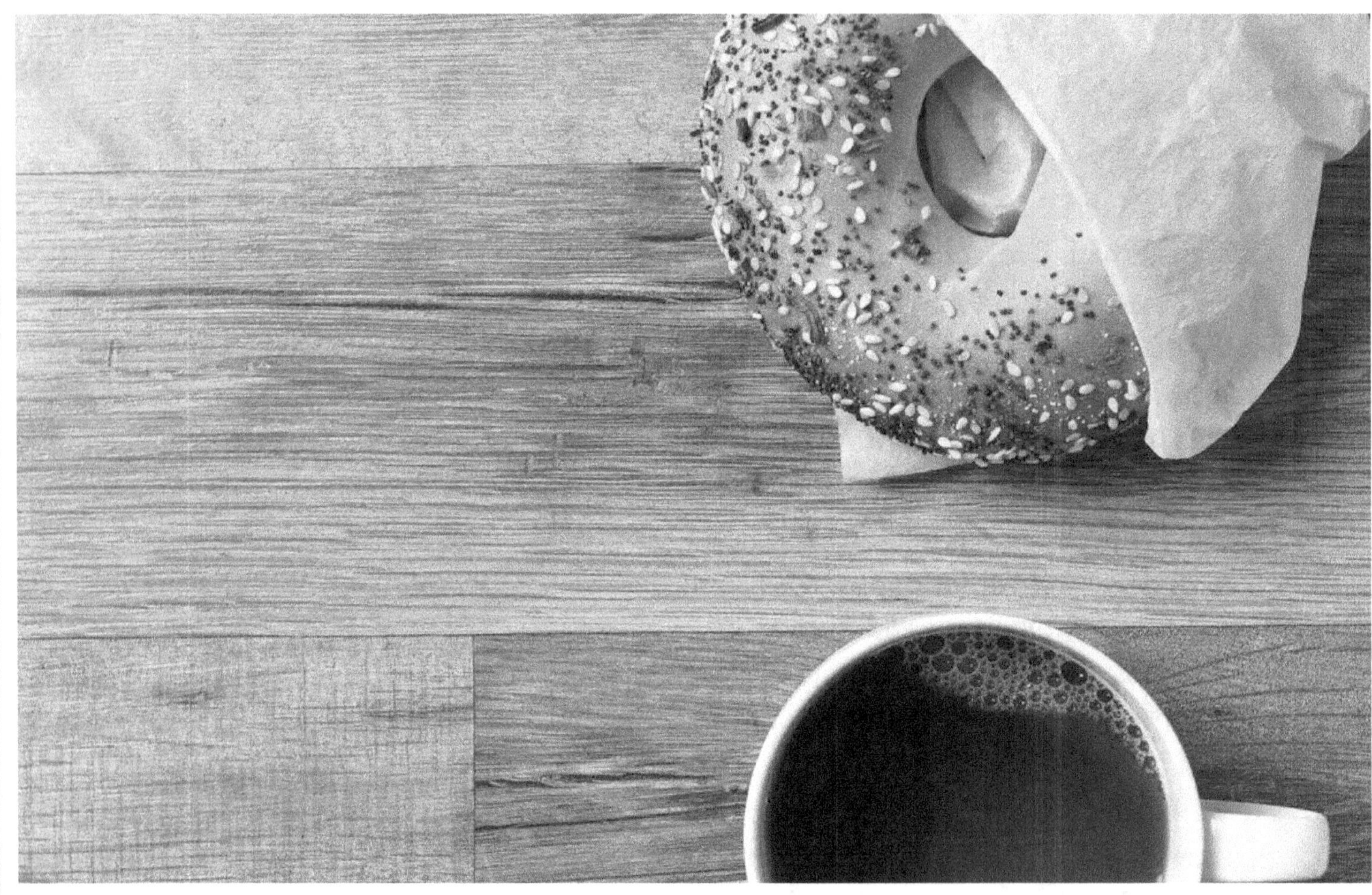

We decided to make use of the fact that we had developed a method for manufacturing structurally and texturally superior bagels, and the San Francisco-style bagel was created.

Nutrition

Calories: 230 | Protein: 8.1g | Fat: 2.2g | Cholesterol: 23.3mg | Sodium: 1323.2mg

Carbohydrates: 43.6g

Ingredients

- 4 cups water
- 1 ¼ cups warm water
- 1 egg, beaten
- 1 tablespoon salt
- 2 teaspoons honey
- 1 pound bread flour, divided in half
- 1 teaspoon cornmeal, or as needed
- 1 ½ teaspoon active dry yeast
- 1 ½ teaspoons salt
- 1 tablespoon sesame seeds, or more if desired

Instructions

1. In the bowl of a stand mixer, combine half of the flour, yeast, and warm water. Cover and set aside at room temperature for thirty minutes or until doubled in size.
2. In the flour-water mixture, add 1 1/2 teaspoons salt and the remaining half of the flour. Knead for about ten minutes with the dough hook of a stand mixer until it forms into a smooth, elastic ball that pulls away from the sides.
3. Remove the dough from the bowl, flour your hands, and gently roll it into a ball. Return to the bowl, cover, and let rise until doubled in size, about one hour fifteen minutes in a warm area.
4. Divide the dough into 8 equal-sized pieces, each weighing about 3 ounces. Make a hole in the center of each piece by stretching it to make an open and even-sized hole.
5. Place on a floured surface, top with more flour, cover with plastic wrap, and set aside for 30 minutes.
6. Preheat the oven to 400 degrees Fahrenheit. Sprinkle a baking sheet with cornmeal.
7. In a large, deep pan, bring 4 cups water, 1 tablespoon salt, and 2 teaspoons, honey to a boil. Boil 2 to 3 bagels in batches for two minutes per side. Allow draining on a wire rack.
8. Place the bagels on the baking sheet that has been prepared. Bake for twenty-five to thirty minutes in a preheated oven until brown and cooked through. Brush with beaten egg and sesame seeds before serving.

PUMPERNICKEL BAGELS

Preparation: 30 Minutes

Cook: 20 Minutes

Servings: 13

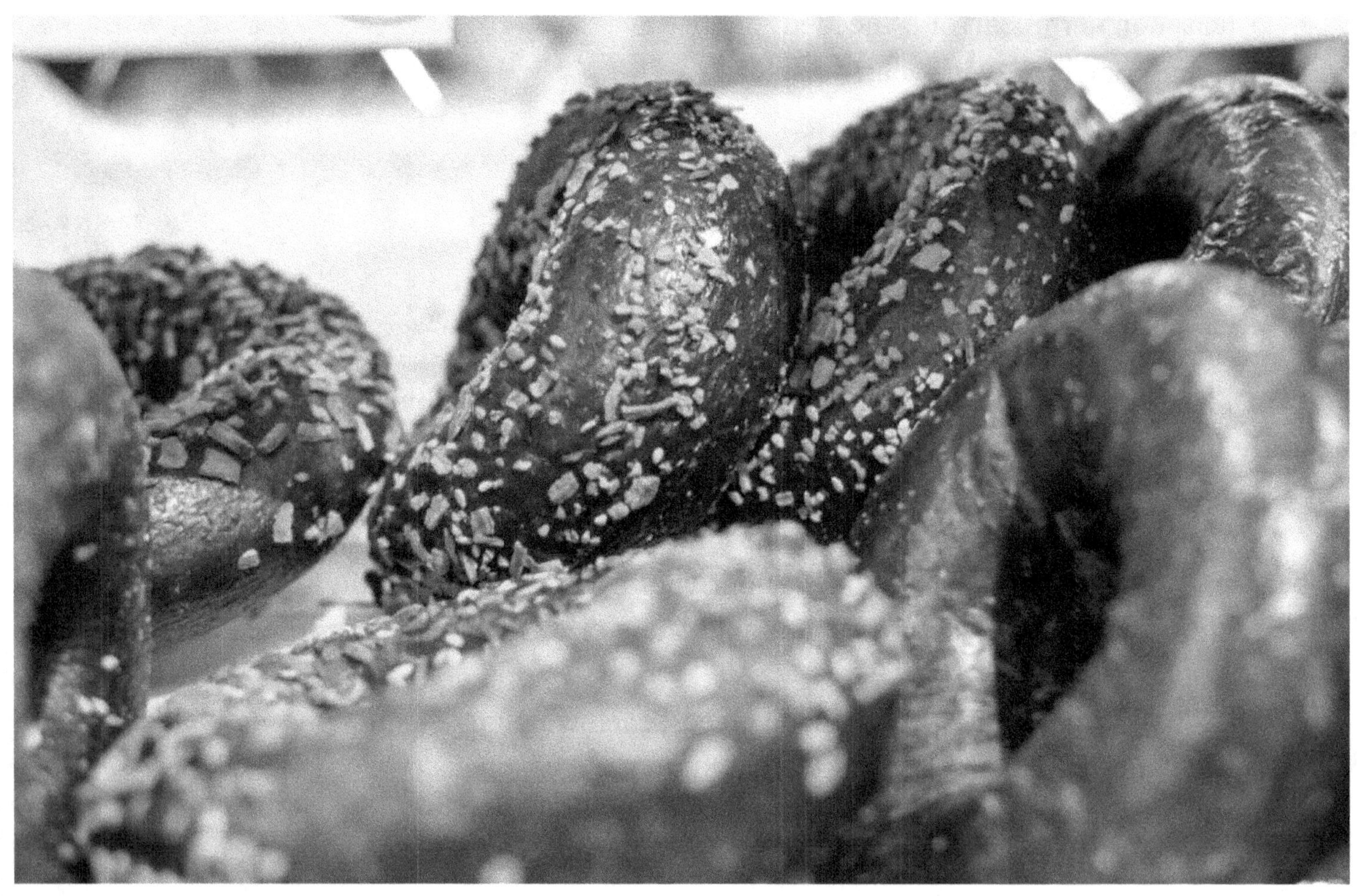

At home, you may make hearty dark rye bagels. These are delicious because they contain rye flour, chocolate, coffee, and caraway seeds.

Nutrition

Calories: 160 | Protein: 4.2g | Fat: 1.9g | Sodium: 284.5mg | Carbohydrates: 33.6g

Ingredients

- 1 cup rye flour
- 1-gallon water
- 1 ¼ cups all-purpose flour
- 4 teaspoons active dry yeast
- ½ cup molasses
- 1 ¼ cups warm water
- ⅓ cup unsweetened cocoa powder
- 1 cup whole-wheat flour
- 1 tablespoon vegetable oil
- 1 tablespoon instant coffee granules
- 1 tablespoon caraway seeds
- 1 ½ teaspoons salt

Instructions

1. In a small mixing bowl, combine warm water, whole-wheat flour, and yeast. Allow 10 minutes for the yeast to soften and begin to foam and bubble.
2. In a large mixing bowl, combine rye flour, molasses, cocoa powder, vegetable oil, coffee granules, caraway seeds, and salt. Combine the yeast mixture and all-purpose flour in a bowl and mix. Turn dough out onto a floured surface and knead for ten minutes, or until smooth and elastic. a slick of grease
3. Cover the dough with a warm wet cloth or plastic wrap and place it in an oiled dish. Allow it to rise in a warm place for 1 hour or until doubled in size.
4. Preheat the oven to 450 degrees Fahrenheit. Grease a baking sheet.
5. In a big pot, bring water to a boil. Divide the dough into 13 pieces and roll each into a ball. Make a hole in the center of each dough ball by pulling the dough to produce a 1-inch hole in the middle while maintaining the dough about 1/2-inch thick. Drop dough circles into boiling water, three or four at a time Cook for forty-five seconds on each side.
6. Bake bagels in the preheated oven until just starting to brown on the bottom, eight to ten minutes.

MULTIGRAIN BAGELS

Preparation: 45 Minutes

Cook: 35 Minutes

Servings: 16

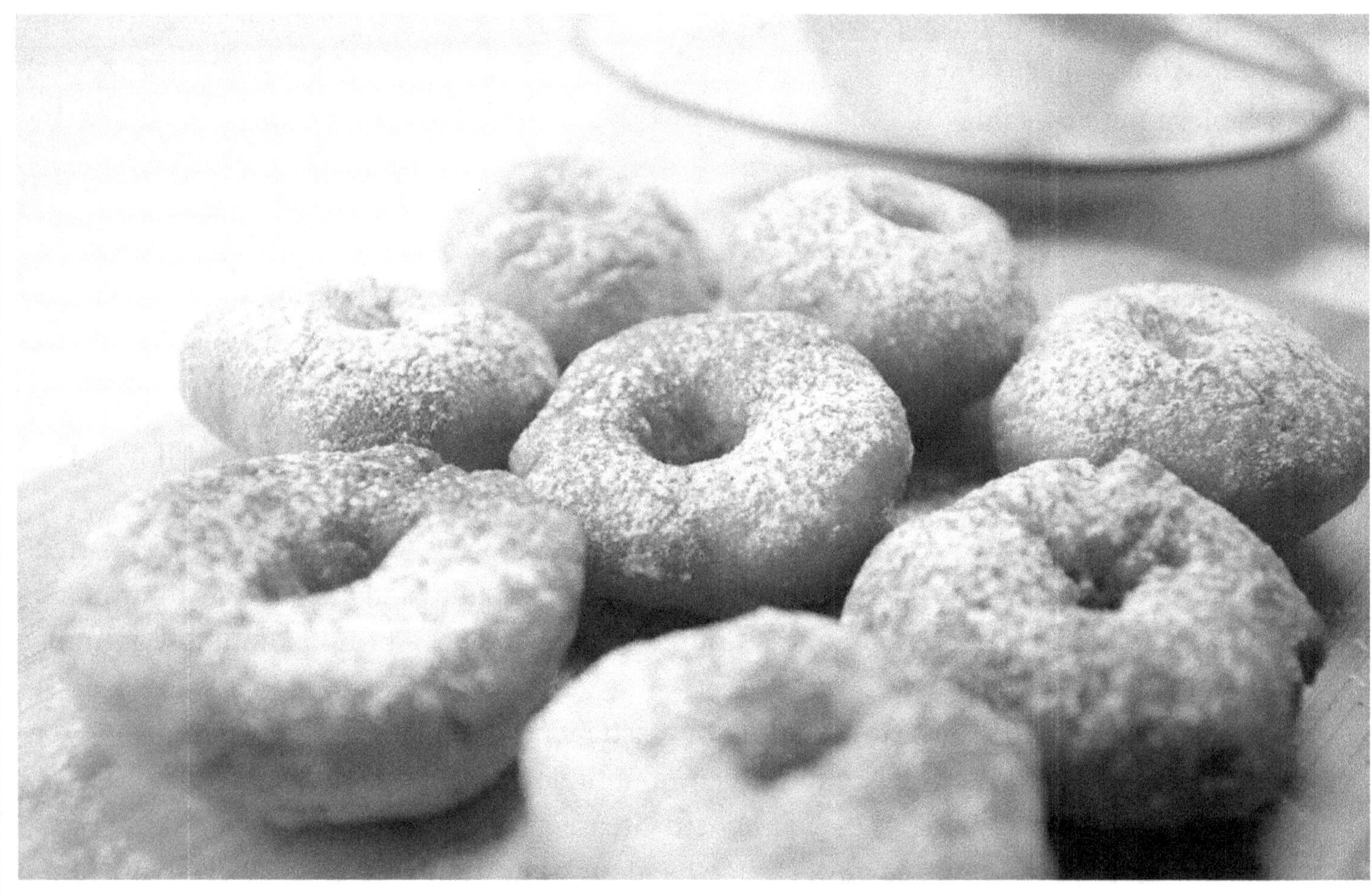

The recipe makes 16 bagels that will not 'go missing' in your toaster. The best way to enjoy these bagels is to toast them. They'll go well with cream cheese and a thin coating of strawberry jam on top. Place in a resealable plastic bag and store.

Nutrition

Calories: 258 | Protein: 10.9g | Fat: 2.6g | Cholesterol: 1.8mg | Sodium: 391.2mg

Carbohydrates: 49.9g

Ingredients

- 1 egg white
- 4 cups whole wheat flour
- 1 cup rolled oats
- ½ teaspoon white sugar
- ¼ cup vital wheat gluten
- ½ cup warm water
- 2 packages of active dry yeast
- 2 cups bread flour
- ¼ cup wheat germ
- 1 ½ tablespoons brown sugar
- 1 tablespoon cornmeal, or as needed
- 3 cups buttermilk
- 3 quarts water
- cooking spray
- 1 teaspoon cool water
- 1 tablespoon sea salt
- ¼ cup organic flaxseed meal
- ⅓ cup orange blossom honey

Instructions

1. In a mixing bowl, combine warm water, yeast, and sugar. Allow 5 minutes for the mixture to dissolve.
2. In a large mixing bowl, combine bread flour, whole wheat flour, rolled oats, vital wheat gluten, wheat germ, flaxseed meal, and salt. Add the buttermilk and mix well. Stir in the yeast mixture and honey until there are no dry spots left. Allow dough to rest for twenty minutes after covering it with plastic wrap.
3. Place the dough on a floured surface. Knead for about seven minutes; it should be soft and sticky. If necessary, add more flour. Make a ball out of it. Using cooking spray, coat a mixing bowl. Turn the dough in the dish to coat it. Cover with plastic wrap and place in a warm, draft-free area for two hours to rise.
4. Preheat the oven to 400 degrees Fahrenheit. Line one 11x17-inch baking sheet with waxed paper, another with a flour sack towel, and the remaining two with cornmeal-dusted parchment paper.
5. In a large pot, combine 3 quarts of water and brown sugar; bring to a boil.

6. Knead the dough briefly on a floured surface. Return one-half of the dough to the bowl and cover. Make a cylinder out of the other half. Cut the dough into quarters and then in half to make 8 equal-sized pieces. Form the dough into balls. Repeat with the remaining dough half.
7. Reduce the heat beneath the sugar-water combination to a low simmer. Cook 2 bagels at a time for thirty seconds on each side in a pot of boiling water. To drain the bagels, place them on a towel-lined baking sheet. Place the bagels on parchment paper-lined baking pans.
8. In a separate dish, whisk together the egg white and 1 teaspoon cool water; use the mixture to brush the tops of the bagels.
9. Preheat the oven to 350°F and bake for twelve minutes. Flip bagels and continue baking until golden brown, about thirty minutes more.
10. Allow it to cool on a wire rack.

BAGEL BREAD

Preparation: 10 Minutes

Cook: 40 Minutes

Servings: 10

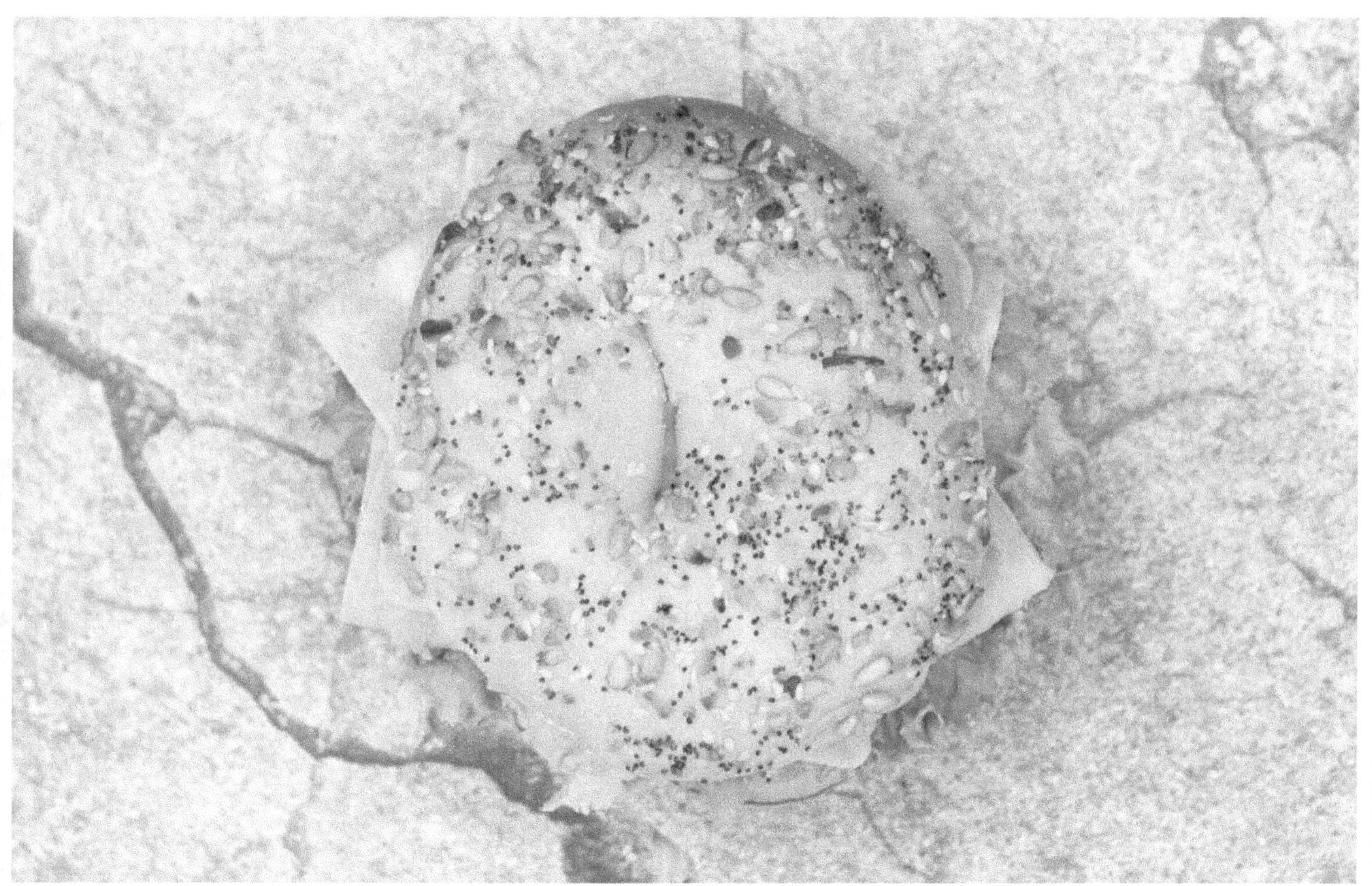

You'll never buy store-bought bread again after you realize how simple it is to create homemade bread in your bread machine

Nutrition

Calories: 20 | Protein: 1.3g | Cholesterol: 19.6mg | Sodium 244.9mg

Carbohydrates: 2.1g | Fat: 0.8g

Ingredients

- 1 egg
- 1 tablespoon white sugar
- 1 ½ teaspoon active dry yeast
- 1 teaspoon salt
- ½ cup milk
- ⅓ cup water
- 2 ¼ cups bread flour

Instructions

1. Place the ingredients in the bread machine pan in the manufacturer's recommended order. Select the Basic White Bread cycle and press the Start button.
2. After the baking cycle is completed, remove the bread from the pan and lay it on a metal rack to cool for one hour before slicing.

NO FAT BANANA BREAD

Preparation: 10 Minutes

Cook: 55 Minutes

Servings: 12

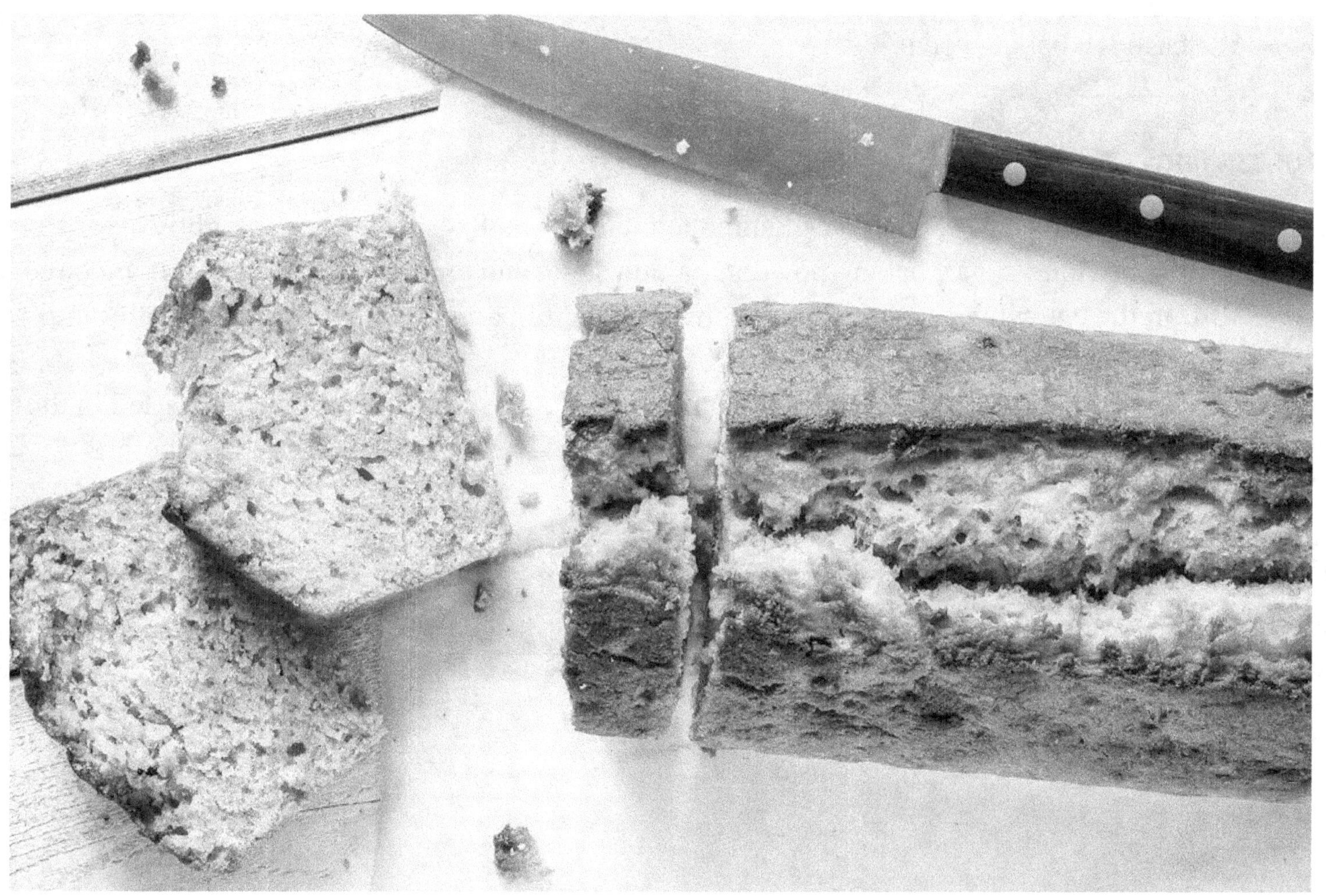

This bread has a fantastic flavor and is surprisingly moist. You can add nuts or raisins for a little extra flavor.

Nutrition

Calories: 127 | Protein: 2.4g | Fat: 0.2g | Sodium: 99.8mg | Carbohydrates: 29.5g

Ingredients

- 2 egg whites
- ¼ cup applesauce
- 1 ¼ teaspoons baking powder
- 1 cup banana, mashed
- ½ teaspoon ground cinnamon
- 1 ½ cups all-purpose flour
- ¾ cup white sugar
- ½ teaspoon baking soda

Instructions

1. Preheat the oven to 350 degrees Fahrenheit. Grease an 8x4-inch loaf pan lightly.
2. Combine flour, sugar, baking powder, baking soda, and cinnamon in a large mixing bowl. Stir in the egg whites, bananas, and applesauce until barely blended. Pour the batter into the pan that has been prepared.
3. Bake for fifty to fifty-five minutes in a preheated oven or until a toothpick inserted in the center of the loaf comes out clean. Allow it to cool completely on a wire rack before slicing.

CHOCOLATE FUDGE BANANA BREAD

Preparation: 10 Minutes

Cook: 1 hr 20 Minutes

Servings: 10

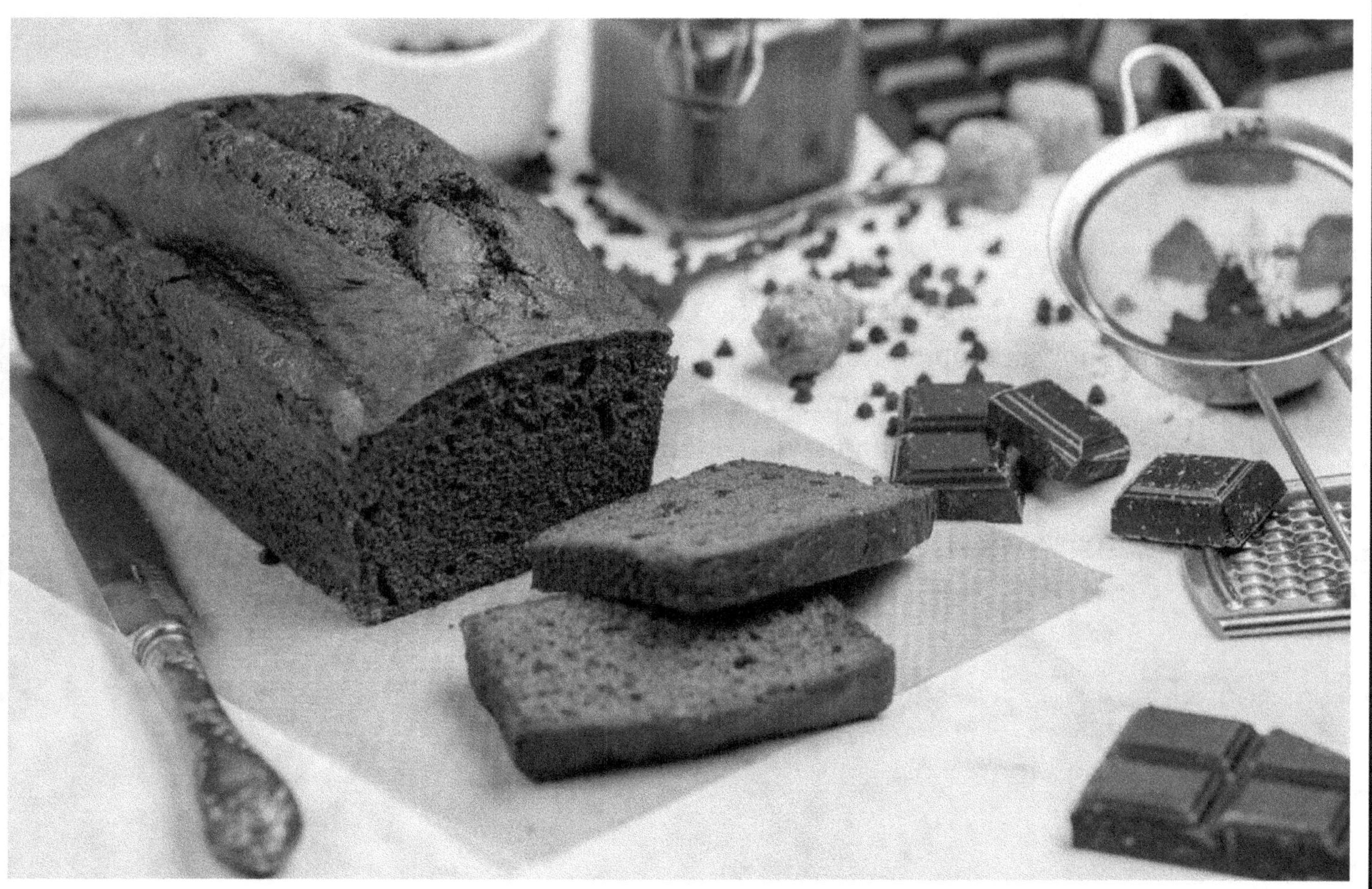

Banana bread that is ooey, gooey, and fudgy. And so delicious, moist, and dense.

Nutrition

Calories: 363 | Protein: 3.7g | Cholesterol: 60mg | Sodium: 318.4mg

Carbohydrates: 47.3g | Fat: 19.1g

Ingredients

- package instant chocolate fudge pudding mix
- 1 cup mashed overripe bananas
- 1 cup miniature milk chocolate chips
- ½ teaspoon salt
- ½ teaspoon baking powder
- large eggs
- ½ cup olive oil
- 1 cup all-purpose flour
- ½ cup white sugar

Instructions

1. Preheat oven to 350 degrees Fahrenheit. Grease a loaf pan and set it aside.
2. In a mixing bowl, combine flour, sugar, pudding mix, salt, and baking powder. Mix the bananas, 3/4 cup chocolate chips, eggs, and oil in a mixing bowl. Pour the mixture into the prepared pan and top with the remaining chocolate chips.
3. Bake for one hour and twenty minutes in a preheated oven or until a toothpick inserted in the center comes out clean.

CREAMY BANANA BREAD

Preparation: 30 Minutes

Cook: 45 Minutes

Servings:16

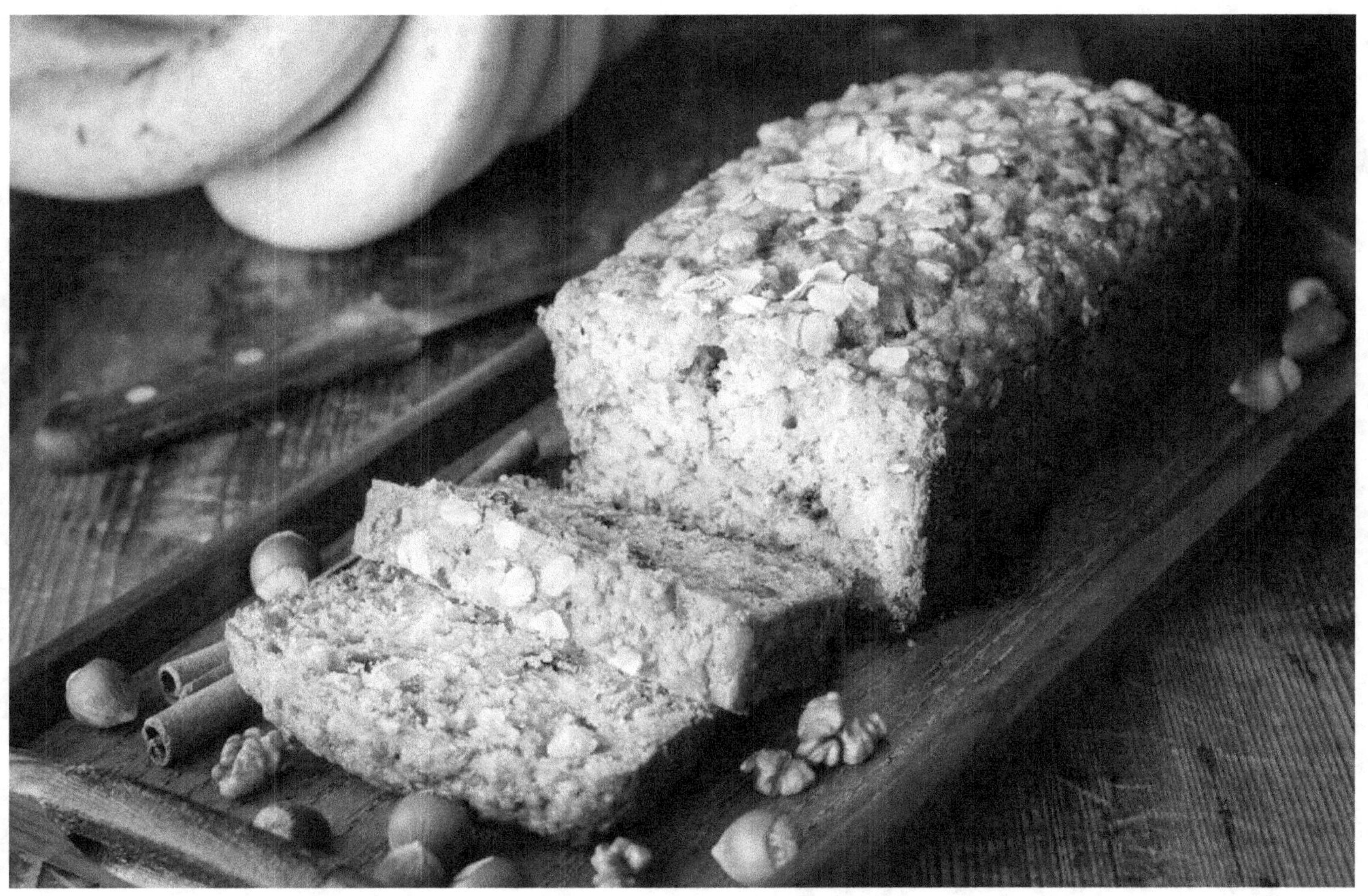

I've been making this recipe for a few years and it's still my family's favourite banana bread! The bananas and cream cheese combine to create this a wonderfully moist bread.

Nutrition

Calories: 289 | Protein: 4.4g | Cholesterol: 38.7mg | Sodium: 212.8mg

Carbohydrates: 35.5g | Fat: 15.1g

Ingredients

- 2 eggs
- 2 ¼ cups all-purpose flour
- ½ cup margarine softened
- ¾ cup chopped pecans
- ½ teaspoon baking soda
- 1 teaspoon vanilla extract
- 2 tablespoons brown sugar
- 2 teaspoons ground cinnamon
- 1 package cream cheese, softened
- 1 ¼ cups white sugar
- 1 cup mashed bananas
- 1 ½ teaspoons baking powder

Instructions

1. Preheat the oven to 350 degrees Fahrenheit. 2 8x4-inch loaf pans, greased and floured
2. Combine the margarine and cream cheese in a mixing bowl. Gradually include the white sugar and beat until light and fluffy. One at a time, add the eggs, beating well after each addition. Combine the mashed bananas and vanilla extract in a mixing bowl. Mix in the flour, baking powder, and baking soda until the batter is just moist.
3. Combine chopped pecans, 2 tablespoons of brown sugar, and cinnamon in a small bowl.
4. Half of the batter goes into each of the two loaf pans. Over the batter in the pans, sprinkle the pecan mixture, then top with the remaining batter.
5. Bake for forty-five minutes in a preheated oven or until a toothpick inserted in the center of each loaf comes out clean.

BANANA PEANUT BUTTER BREAD

Preparation: 15 Minutes

Cook: 1 hr 10 Minutes

Servings: 15

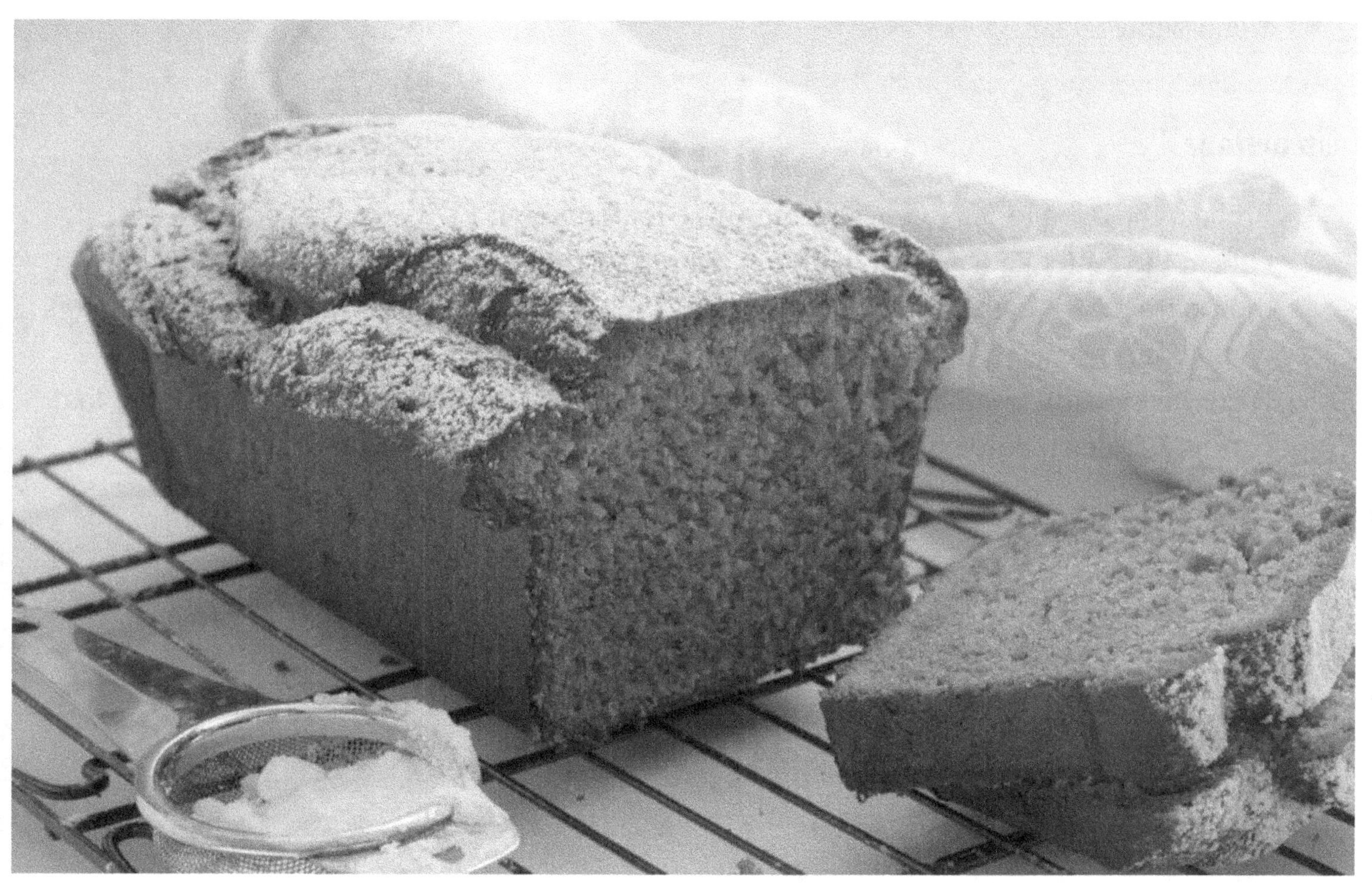

Quick, simple, and delicious. It's great for breakfast or as a snack.

Nutrition

Calories: 266 | Protein: 5.5g | Fat: 13.9g | Cholesterol: 41.1mg | Sodium: 179.2mg

Carbohydrates: 32.1g

Ingredients

- 2 eggs
- 2 cups all-purpose flour 2 bananas, mashed
- ½ cup peanut butter
- 1 teaspoon baking soda
- ½ cup chopped walnuts
- ½ cup butter softened
- 1 cup white sugar

Instructions

1. Preheat the oven to 325. Grease a 5x9-inch loaf pan lightly.
2. Cream the butter and sugar together in a large mixing dish. Add the eggs and beat them thoroughly. Mix in the peanut butter, bananas, flour, and baking soda until everything is well combined. Toss in the walnuts. Pour into the pan that has been prepared.
3. Bake for seventy minutes at 325°F, or until a toothpick inserted in the center of the loaf comes out clean. Allow it to cool on a wire rack.

BANANA CRUMB MUFFINS

Preparation: 15 Minutes

Cook: 20 Minutes

Servings: 10

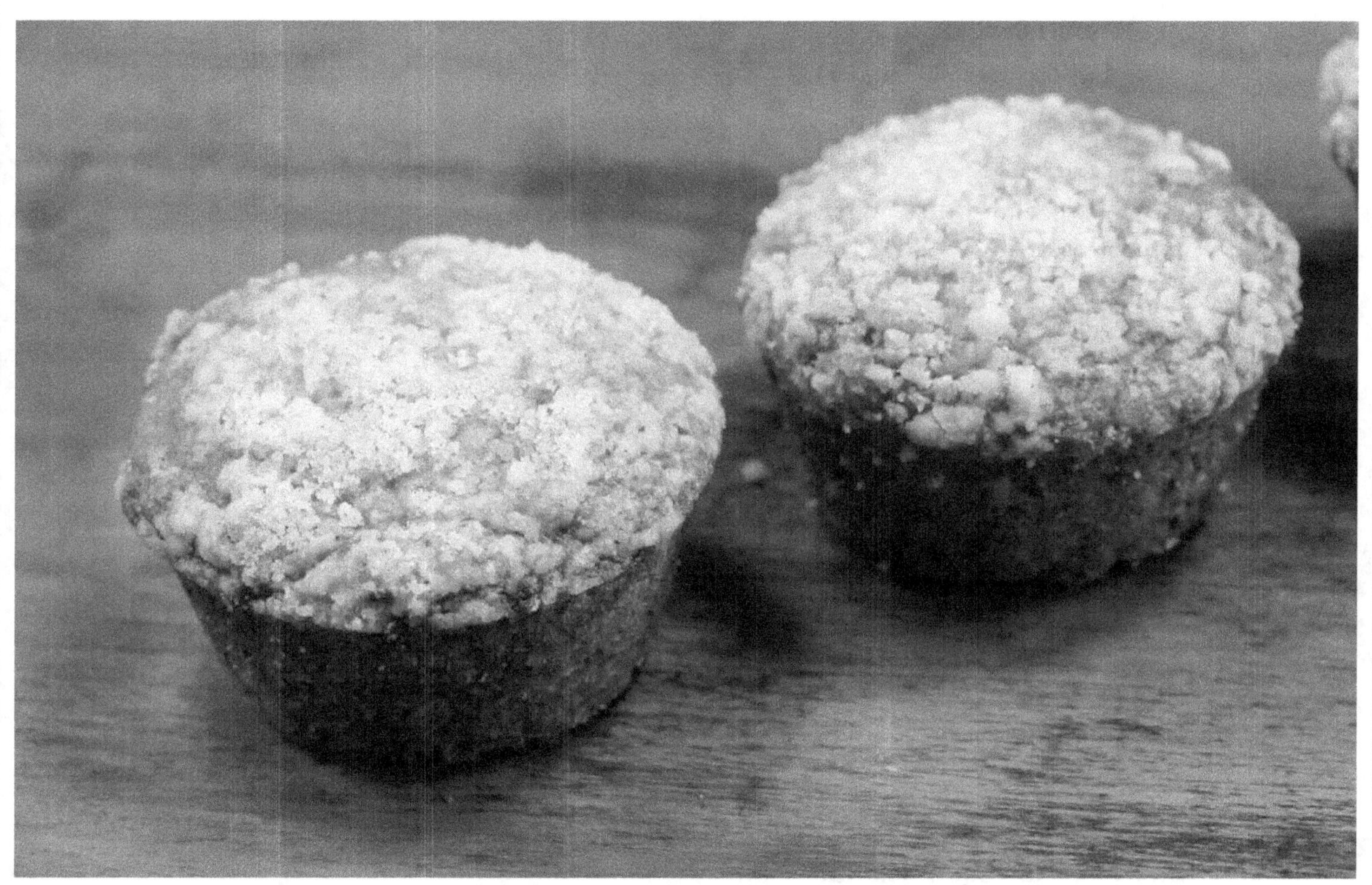

The crumb topping is what distinguishes these banana muffins from the rest. They're delicious

Nutrition

Calories: 263 | Protein: 3.2g | Cholesterol: 37.9mg | Sodium 352.5mg

Carbohydrates: 46g | Fat: 8.1g

Ingredients

- 1 egg, lightly beaten
- 2 tablespoons all-purpose flour
- 3 bananas, mashed
- ⅓ cup packed brown sugar
- 1 tablespoon butter
- ⅛ teaspoon ground cinnamon
- 1 ½ cups all-purpose flour
- 1 teaspoon baking soda
- 1 teaspoon baking powder
- ½ teaspoon salt
- ¾ cup white sugar
- ⅓ cup butter, melted

Instructions

1. Preheat the oven to 375 degrees Fahrenheit. Ten muffin cups will be lightly greased or lined with muffin papers.
2. Combine 1 1/2 cups flour, baking soda, baking powder, and salt in a large mixing dish. Combine bananas, sugar, egg, and melted butter in a separate bowl. Just until the flour mixture is moistened, stir in the banana mixture. Fill muffin cups halfway with batter.
3. Combine brown sugar, 2 tablespoons flour, and cinnamon in a small bowl. 1 tablespoon butter, cut in until mixture resembles coarse cornmeal. Sprinkle the topping on top of the muffins.
4. Bake for eighteen to twenty minutes in a preheated oven or until a toothpick inserted in the center of a muffin comes out clean.

BANANA-NUT MINI LOAVES WITH CHOCOLATE CHIPS

Preparation: 15 Minutes

Cook: 25 Minutes

Servings: 16

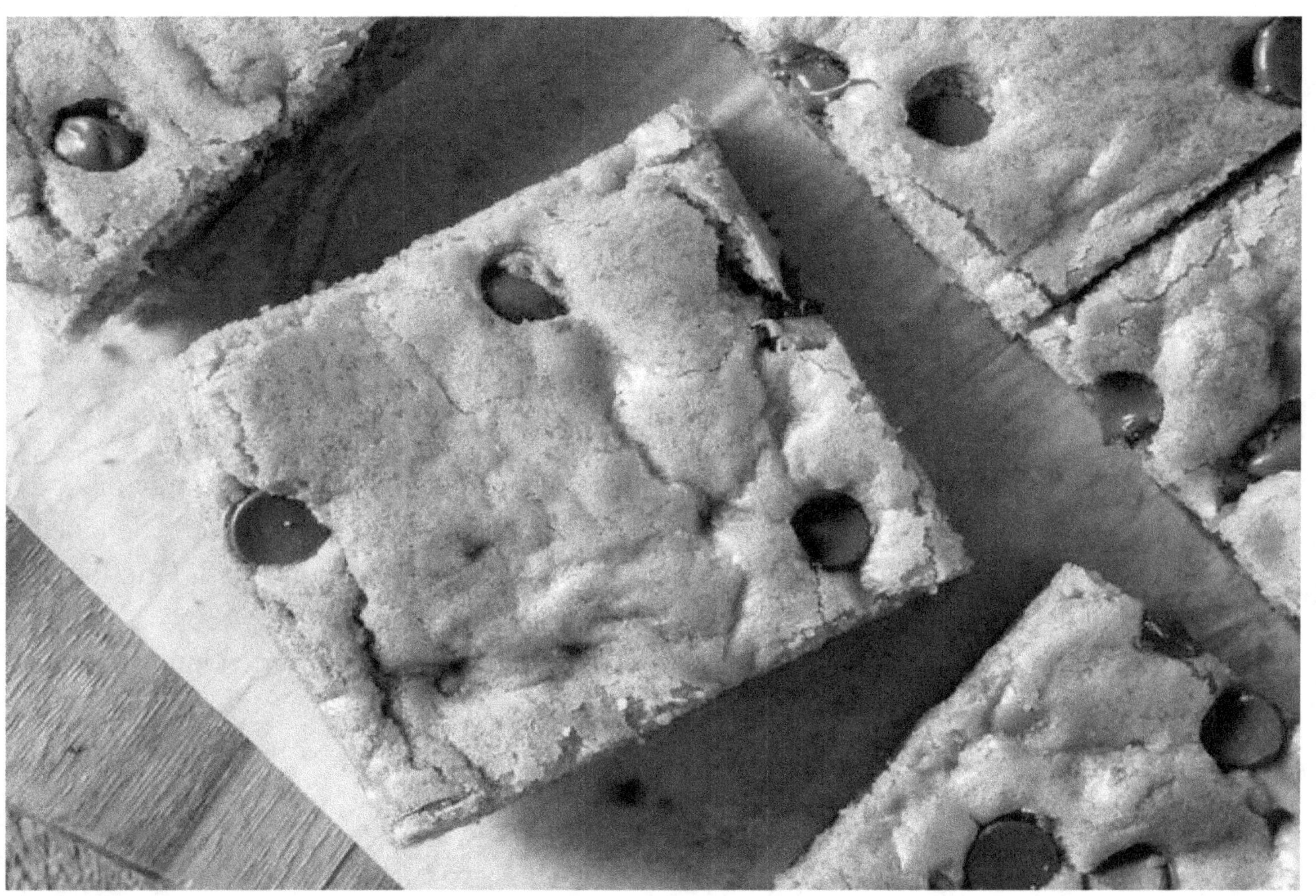

Banana bread mini loaves with walnuts and chocolate chips.

Nutrition

Calories: 201 | Protein: 3.9g | Cholesterol: 11.6mg | Sodium: 140.2mg

Carbohydrates: 35.1g | Fat: 6.6g

Ingredients

- cooking spray
- 1 large egg
- 2 cups whole wheat flour
- 1 teaspoon baking soda
- ¾ cup semisweet chocolate chips
- ½ teaspoon ground cinnamon
- 1 teaspoon vanilla extract
- 3 very ripe bananas, mashed
- 1 cup white sugar
- ½ teaspoon sea salt
- ½ cup unsweetened applesauce
- ¾ cup chopped walnuts

Instructions

1. Preheat the oven to 350°F. Using cooking spray, coat an 8-count mini loaf pan.
2. With a wooden spoon, combine the sugar, applesauce, egg, and vanilla in a large mixing dish. Stir in the bananas, walnuts, and chocolate chips until everything is well combined. Stir in the flour, baking soda, cinnamon, and salt until thoroughly combined. Pour the batter into the loaf pan that has been prepared.
3. Bake for twenty-five to thirty minutes, or until a toothpick or fork inserted into the center comes out clean. Allow at least thirty minutes for cooling.

EXTREME BANANA NUT BREAD

Preparation: 15 Minutes

Cook: 20 Minutes

Servings: 10

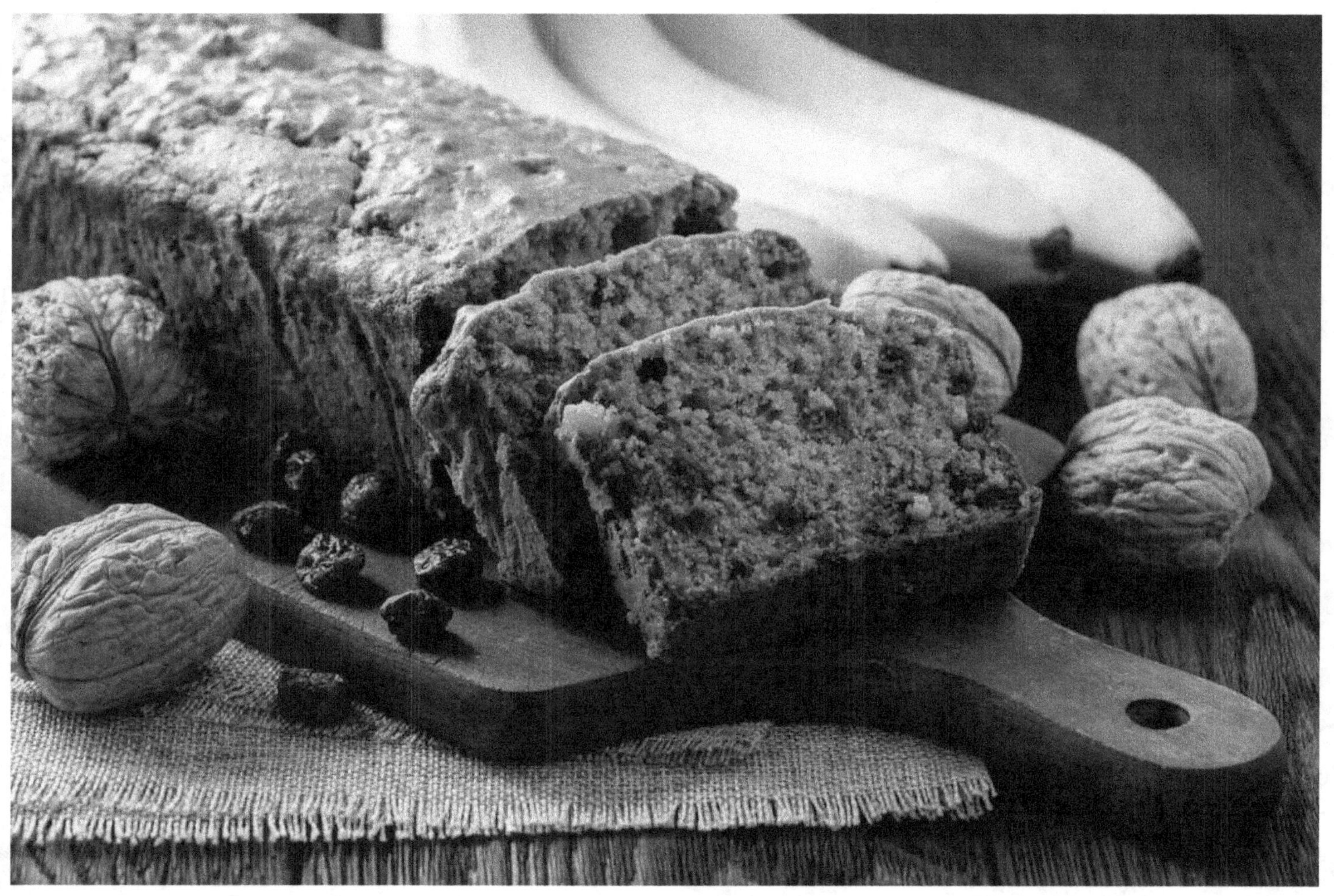

This is a fairly adaptable recipe that will work with anything you have on hand. In place of butter, use any sort of fat, such as shortening or oil. It also works with brown or white sugar.

Nutrition

Calories: 232 | Protein: 3.2g | Cholesterol: 51.3mg | Sodium: 268.4mg

Carbohydrates: 29.7g | Fat: 11.9g

Ingredients

- 4 eggs, beaten
- 2 cups all-purpose flour
- 2 teaspoons baking soda
- 1 cup chopped walnuts
- 2 cups white sugar
- 2 cups mashed overripe bananas
- 1 teaspoon salt
- 1 cup butter or margarine

Instructions

1. Preheat the oven to 350°F . 2 9x5 inch loaf pans, greased and floured
2. In a large mixing dish, sift together the flour, salt, and baking soda. Mix the butter or margarine and sugar in a separate bowl until smooth. In a large mixing bowl, combine the bananas, eggs, and walnuts until well combined. Pour the wet ingredients into the dry ingredients and whisk just until everything is combined. Evenly distribute the batter between the two loaf pans.
3. In a preheated oven, bake for sixty to seventy minutes, or until a knife inserted into the crown of the loaf comes out clean. Allow at least five minutes for the loaves to cool in the pans before turning out onto a cooling rack to cool entirely. To keep the moisture in, wrap it in aluminum foil. Refrigerate the loaves for at least two hours before serving.

EINKORN BANANA BREAD

Preparation: 20 Minutes

Cook: 55 Minutes

Servings: 12

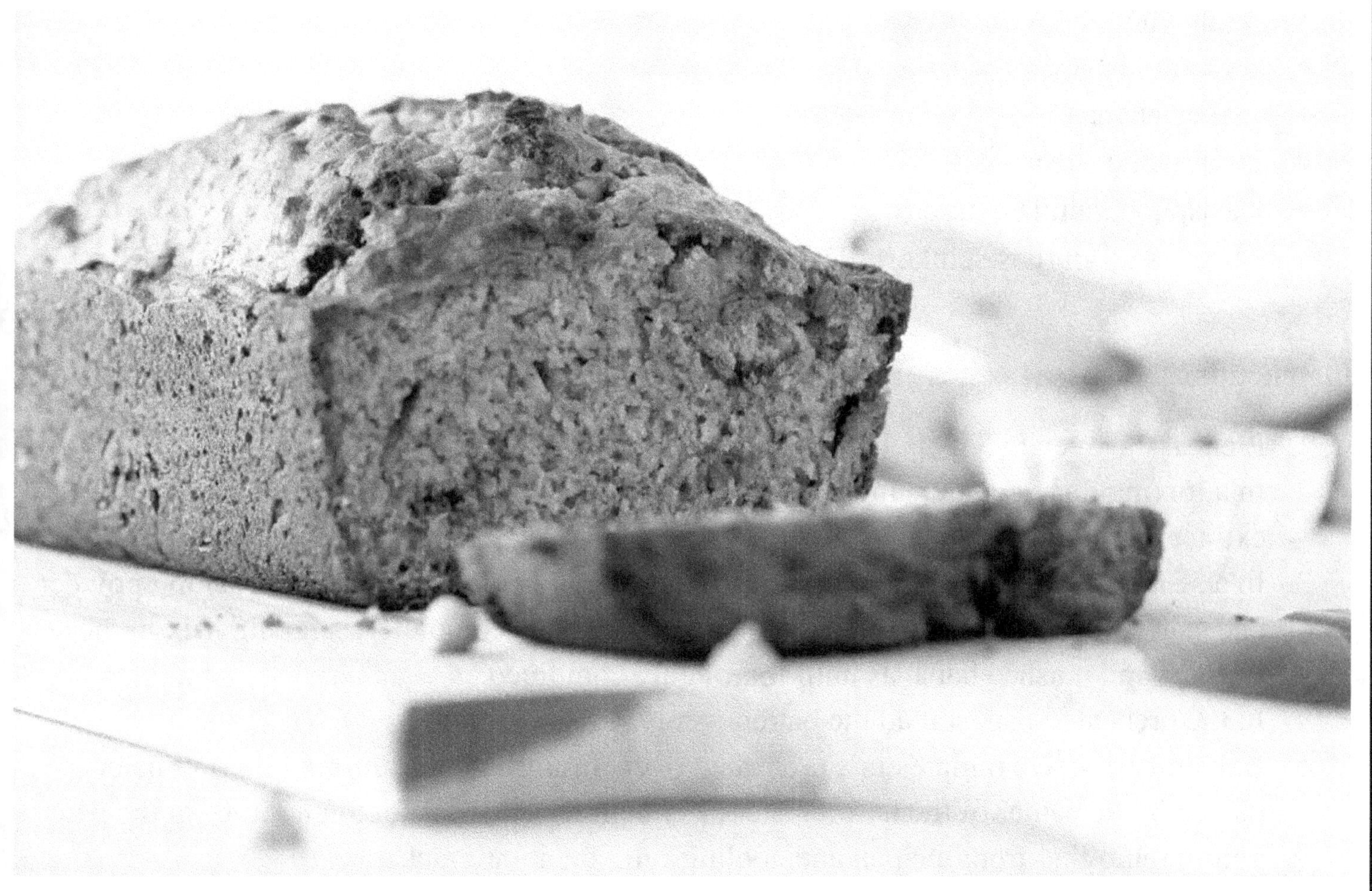

Using einkorn wheat in your banana bread will add extra nutrients and protein. Einkorn flour is equally as adaptable as all-purpose flour and can be used in place of it cup for cup. The flavor will take your breath away.

Nutrition

Calories: 255 | Protein: 4.2g | Cholesterol: 51.4mg | Sodium: 261.1mg

Carbohydrates: 34.5g | Fat: 14.3g

Ingredients

- 2 eggs
- 1 tablespoon milk
- ½ cup butter, melted
- 1 teaspoon baking powder
- 1 teaspoon ground cinnamon
- 1 teaspoon baking soda
- ½ cup chopped walnuts
- ¼ teaspoon salt
- 3 ripe bananas
- 1 cup white sugar
- 1 teaspoon vanilla extract
- 1 ½ cups all-purpose einkorn flour, sifted

Instructions

1. Preheat the oven to 350°F. Using butter, grease a 9x5-inch loaf pan.
2. In a mixing dish, combine melted butter and sugar. Mix in the eggs, milk, and vanilla extract thoroughly.
3. In a separate bowl, combine sifted einkorn flour, cinnamon, baking soda, baking powder, and salt. Stir the flour into the butter mixture until it is completely smooth. Mix in the walnuts and mashed bananas until thoroughly combined.
4. In the preheated pan, spread the batter evenly.
5. Bake for fifty-five minutes in a preheated oven, or until an instant-read thermometer placed in the center of the loaf registers 195 degrees F . Cool for ten minutes in the pan before removing from the pan and cooling fully on a wire rack.

BANANA OATMEAL BREAD

Preparation: 15 Minutes

Cook: 1 hr 5 Minutes

Servings: 12

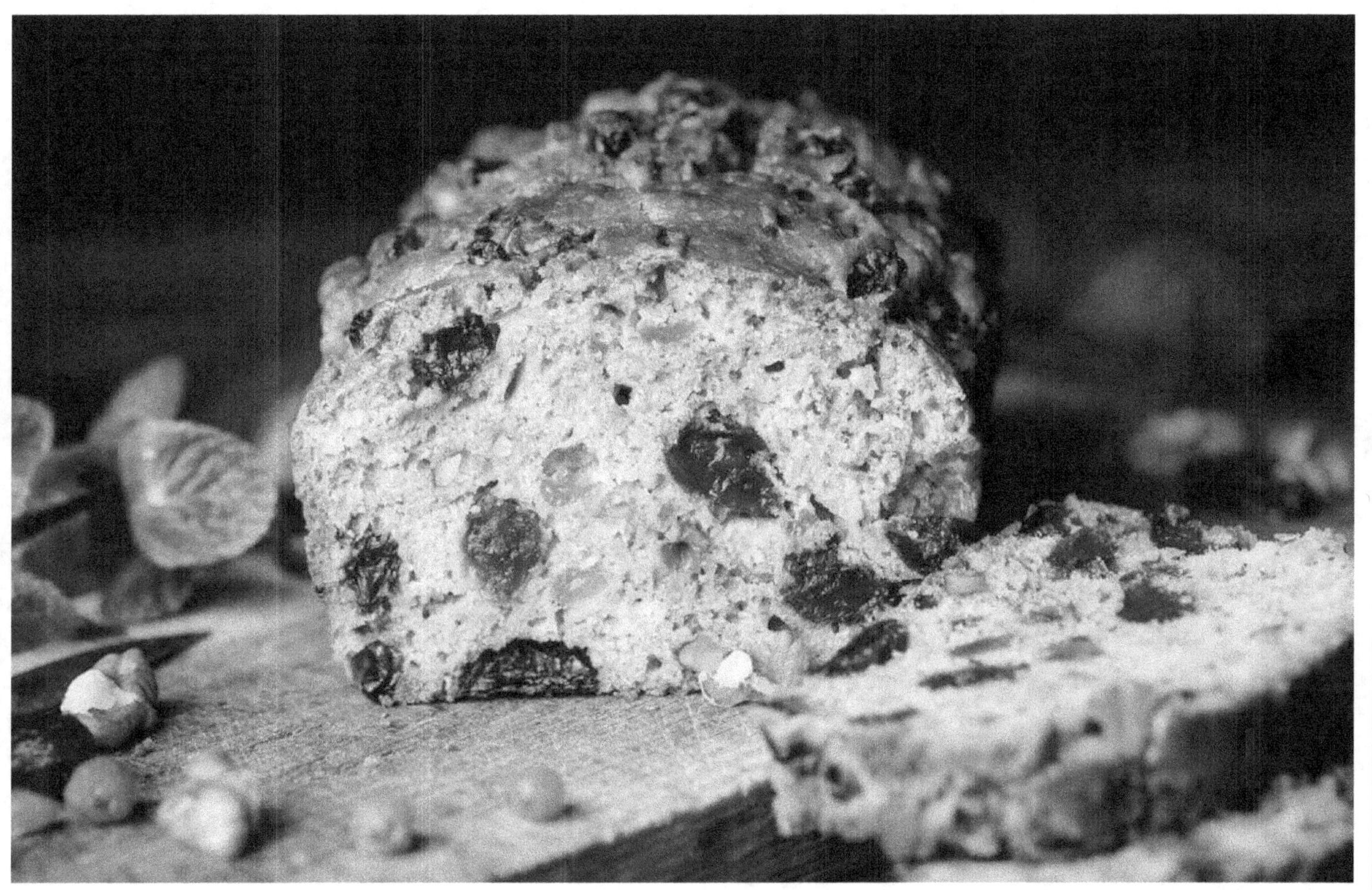

This is an old family dish that is moist and delicious.

Nutrition

Calories: 229 | Protein: 3.8g | Cholesterol: 51.3mg | Sodium: 222.9mg

Carbohydrates: 34.8g | Fat: 8.8g

Ingredients

- 1 cup all-purpose flour
- 2 eggs, beaten
- ¼ cup milk
- ½ teaspoon ground cinnamon
- ½ cup shortening
- 1 teaspoon baking soda
- ½ teaspoon salt
- 1 ½ cups mashed bananas
- 1 cup white sugar
- ½ teaspoon vanilla extract
- 1 cup quick-cooking oats
- ½ cup chopped raisins (optional)

Instructions

1. Preheat the oven to 350 degrees Fahrenheit. Set aside a 9x5-inch loaf pan that has been greased.
2. Mix the shortening and sugar in a mixing bowl. Beat in the eggs and vanilla extract until light and frothy.
3. Combine the flour, oatmeal, baking soda, salt, and cinnamon in a sifter. Alternate adding dry ingredients with bananas and milk. Mix until everything is well combined.
4. Preheat oven to 350°F and bake for fifty-sixty minutes. Pour into the prepared pan after folding in the raisins. Remove from oven and set aside for five minutes.

BANANA COCONUT LOAF

Preparation: 15 Minutes

Cook: 20 Minutes

Servings: 10

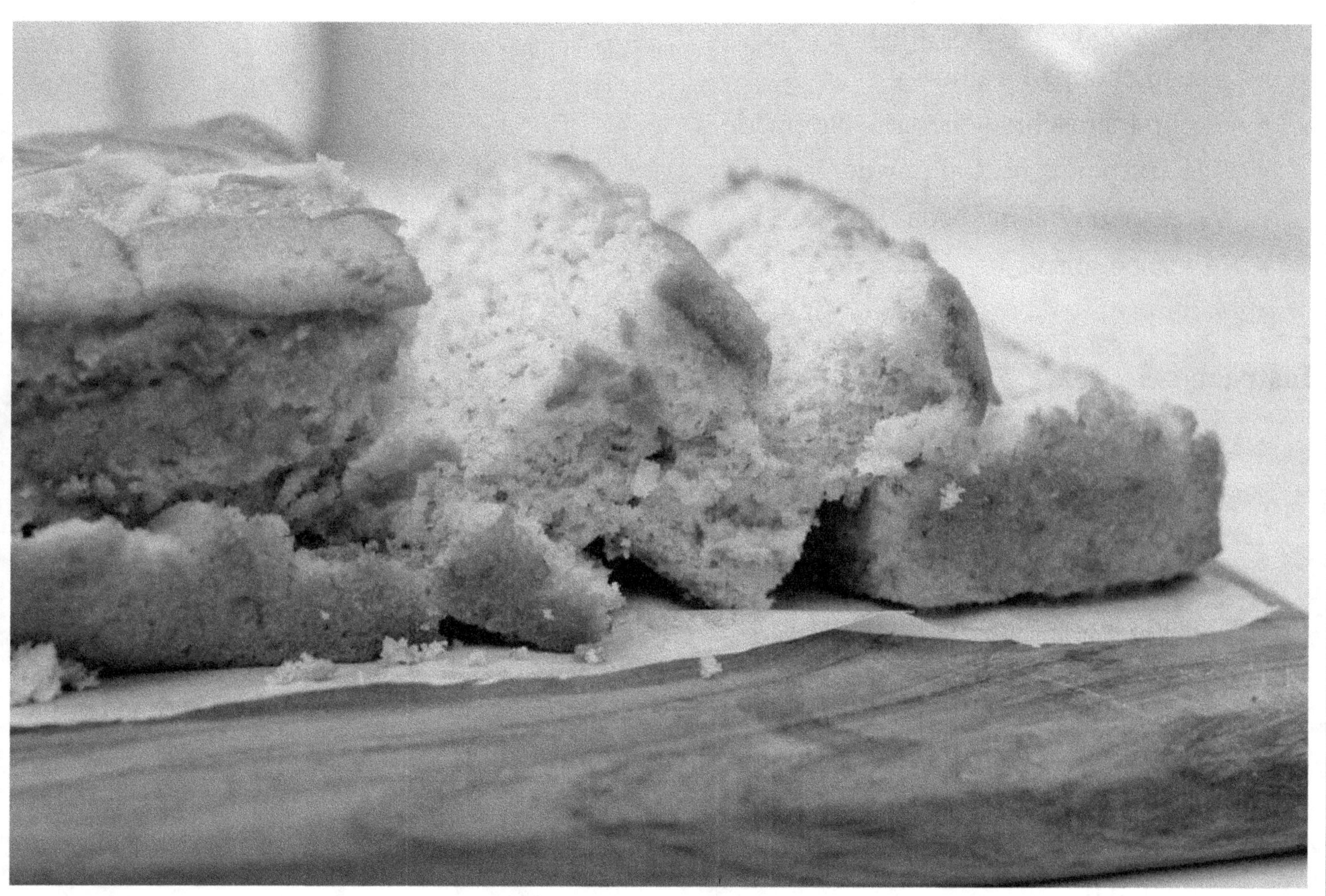

A beautiful loaf with a flavor to match.

Nutrition

Calories: 264 | Protein: 3.7g | Fat: 10.1g | Cholesterol: 31.4mg | Sodium: 217.2mg

Carbohydrates: 41.5g

Ingredients

- 2 eggs
- ½ cup flaked coconut
- ½ cup butter, melted
- 1 ½ cups all-purpose flour
- 1 cup white sugar
- 1 cup mashed bananas
- ½ teaspoon almond extract
- ½ cup chopped walnuts
- ½ cup maraschino cherries, chopped
- 1 ½ teaspoons baking powder
- ½ teaspoon baking soda
- ½ teaspoon salt

Instructions

1. Combine flour, coconut, baking powder, baking soda, salt, walnuts, and cherries in a mixing bowl.
2. In a mixing dish, crack the eggs and whisk them until light and foamy. Mix the sugar and melted butter or margarine in a mixing bowl. Beat the drums thoroughly. Put the mashed banana and seasoning in a mixing bowl. Stir in the flour mixture until it is completely combined. Fill a greased 9x5x3-inch loaf pan halfway with batter.
3. Bake for one hour at 350°F/175°C, or until a toothpick inserted in the center comes out clean. Allow it to cool for ten minutes before removing from pan. Cool.

APPLE CIDER-CRANBERRY BREAD

Preparation: 15 Minutes

Cook: 40 Minutes

Servings: 10

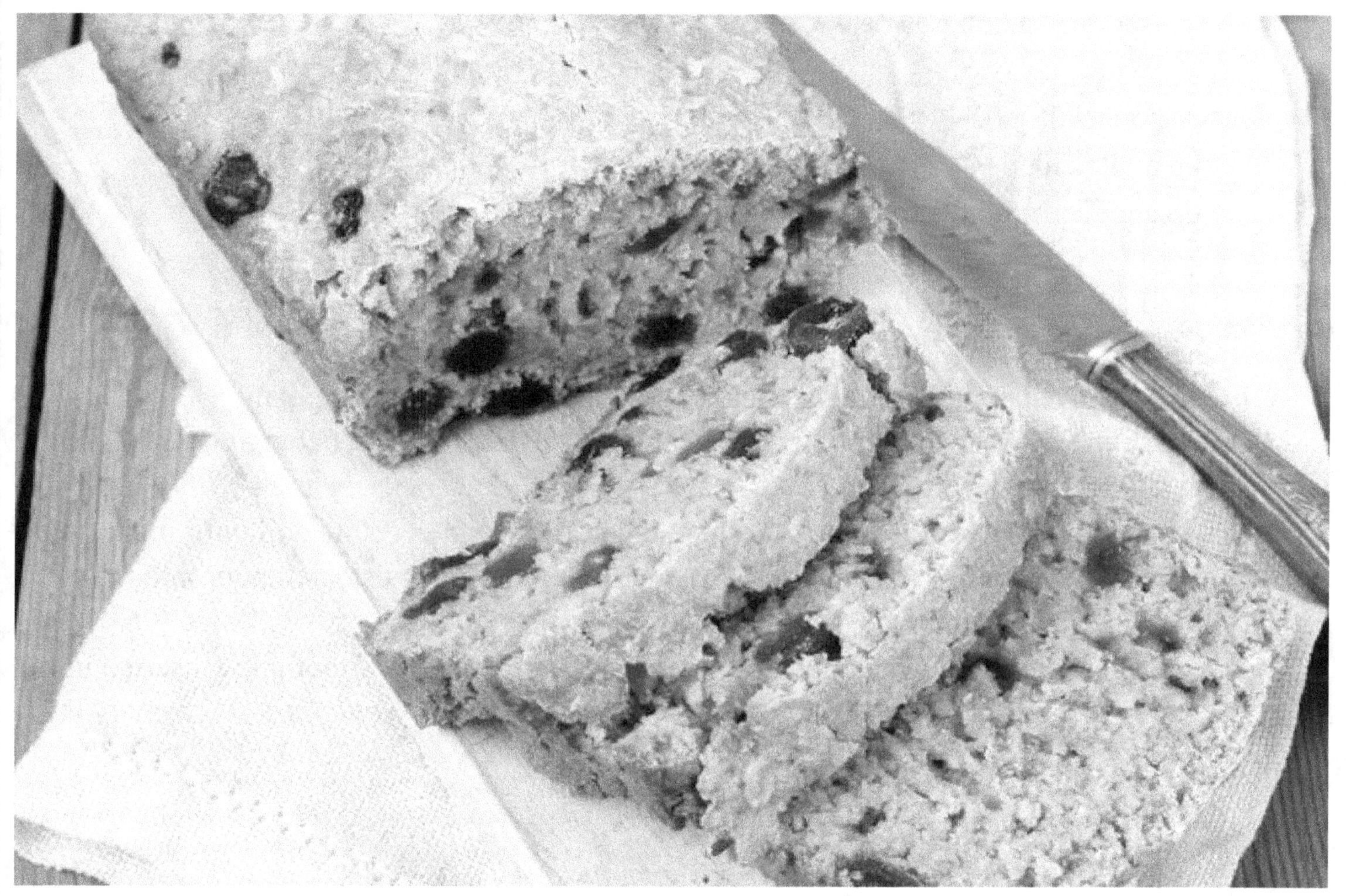

This apple cider bread is sweet and slightly acidic, perfect for breakfast, snacking, or whenever you need a little something. Good luck with your baking.

Nutrition

Calories: 281 | Protein: 5g | Cholesterol: 32.7mg | Sodium: 267.4mg

Carbohydrates: 45.4g | Fat: 9.6g

Ingredients

- cooking spray
- 2 eggs
- ⅛ cup vegetable oil
- 2 cups all-purpose flour
- ¾ cup dried cranberries
- ½ teaspoon baking soda
- 1 ½ teaspoons baking powder
- ¾ cup white sugar
- ½ teaspoon salt
- ¾ cup apple cider
- ¾ cup chopped walnuts (optional)

Instructions

1. Preheat the oven to 350°F. Using cooking spray, coat a 9x5-inch loaf pan.
2. In a large mixing dish, combine flour, sugar, cranberries, walnuts, baking powder, baking soda, and salt.
3. In a second bowl, whisk together the apple cider, eggs, and vegetable oil until foamy. Mix the apple cider mixture into the flour mixture until it is moistened; pour into the loaf pan that has been prepared.
4. Bake for forty to forty-five minutes in a preheated oven or until a toothpick inserted in the center comes out clean.

CRANBERRY PECAN BREAD

Preparation: 30 Minutes

Cook:1 hr 15 Minutes

Servings:12

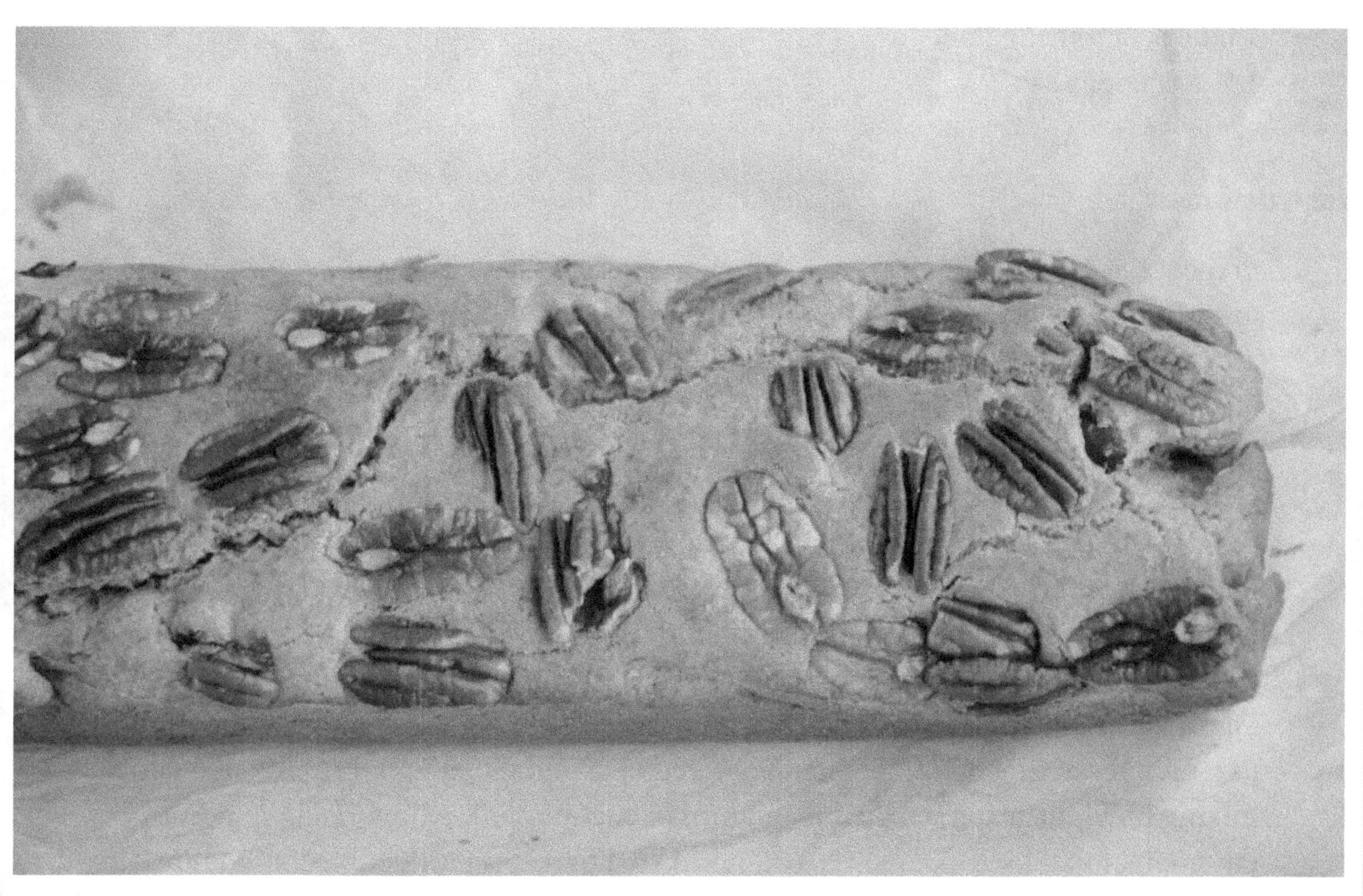

Dried cranberries and pecans are mixed into a simple sourdough starter-fermented loaf. We like to use it to make French toast.

Nutrition

Calories: 219 | Protein: 5.3g | Cholesterol: 2.6mg | Sodium: 302.3mg

Carbohydrates: 35.8g | Fat: 6.4g

Ingredients

- 1 cup water
- 1 ½ cups all-purpose flour
- ¾ cup dried cranberries
- 1 ½ cups bread flour
- ¾ cup sourdough starter
- ¾ cup coarsely chopped pecans
- 1 tablespoon melted butter
- 1 ½ teaspoons salt

Instructions

1. Preheat the oven to 275 degrees Fahrenheit. Spread the pecans out on a baking sheet and toast for forty-five minutes, or until they turn golden brown and fragrant. When the nuts are baking, keep an eye on them because they can burn rapidly. Set the nuts aside to cool once they've been toasted.
2. While you're creating the dough, cover the cranberries with hot water and let them soak.
3. In the bowl of a stand mixer or a mixing bowl, combine the all-purpose flour and bread flour with the water to produce a rough dough. Allow thirty minutes to rest after covering the bowl with plastic wrap.
4. Knead in the sourdough starter and salt until the dough is smooth and elastic, three to five minutes if using a stand mixer, or nine to eleven minutes if doing it by hand.
5. Drain the cranberries and mix them with the pecans in the dough. Knead for another one-two minutes to properly integrate the ingredients into the dough. Lightly oil a large mixing bowl, then add the dough and turn to coat it in oil. Allow rising in a warm environment 80 to 95 degrees F for four to six hours, or until doubled in volume.
6. Do not knead the dough. Form a round loaf out of the risen dough on a lightly floured work surface. Allow for a ten-minute rest period. Form the dough into a round or oblong loaf, set it on parchment paper, dust it lightly with flour, and let it rise for another one to two hours, or until about doubled in size.
7. Preheat the oven to 400 degrees Fahrenheit. Allow at least forty-five minutes for a baking or pizza stone to heat in the oven before baking.
8. Brush the top of the loaf with water, and use a sharp knife to make shallow incisions in the loaf. Place the loaf and parchment paper on top of a baking sheet or stone in the oven and bake for thirty to thirty-five minutes, or until the loaf is golden brown and hollow when tapped. Place the loaf on a cooling rack and brush with melted butter before slicing.

CRANBERRY LOAF

Preparation: 15 Minutes

Cook: 20 Minutes

Servings: 10

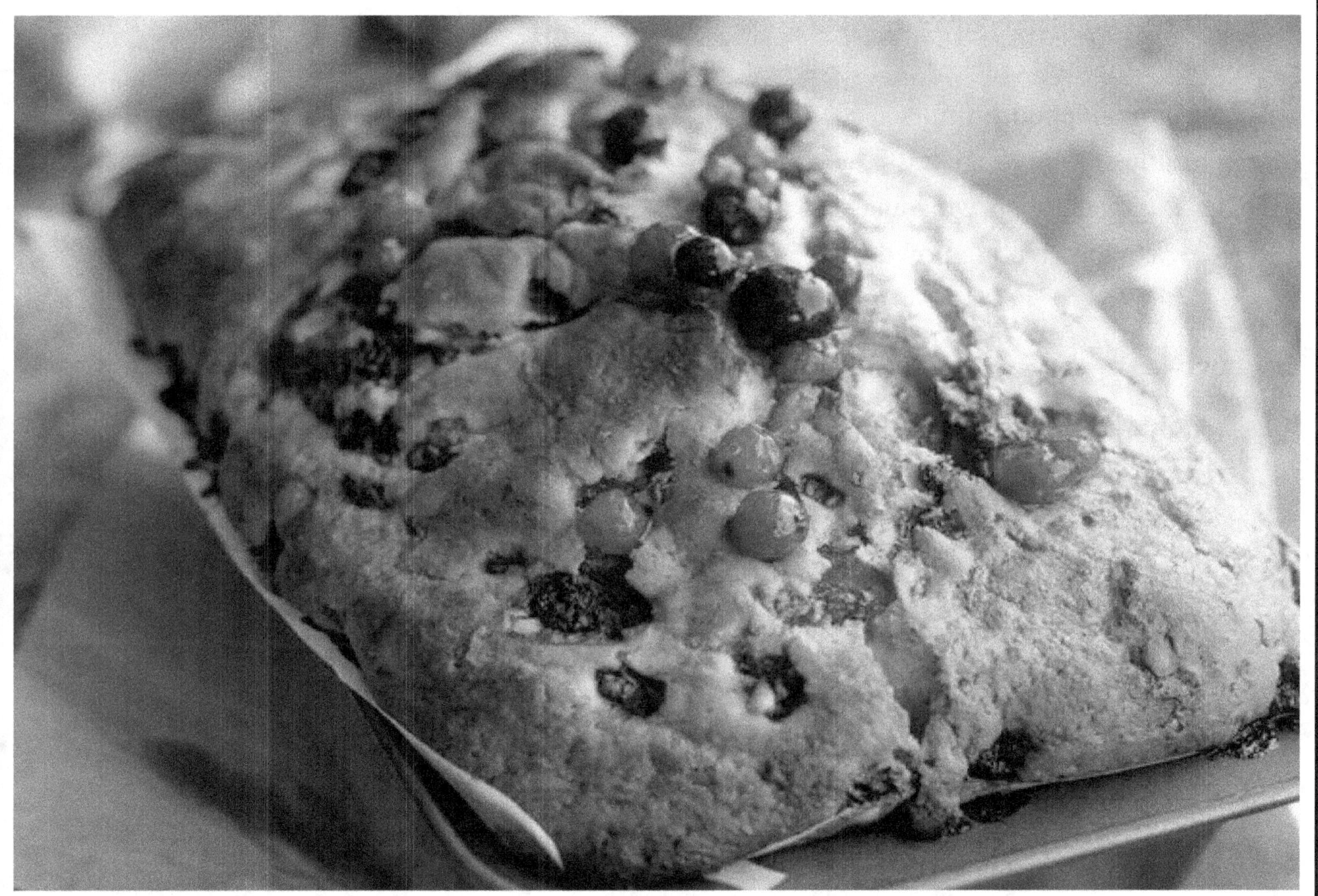

You'll almost wish you had more of this bread because it's almost acidic.

Nutrition

Calories: 245 | Protein: 3.4g | Fat: 10.6g | Cholesterol: 15.5mg | Sodium: 231mg

Carbohydrates: 36.2g

Ingredients

- 1 egg, beaten
- 1 cup orange juice
- 1 cup raisins
- ½ teaspoon salt
- ⅓ cup vegetable oil
- 1 cup all-purpose flour
- 1 cup chopped cranberries
- 1 cup graham cracker crumbs
- ½ cup chopped walnuts
- 1 tablespoon orange zest
- ½ cup packed brown sugar
- 2 teaspoons baking powder

Instructions

1. Combine flour, crumbs, brown sugar, baking powder, and salt in a large mixing bowl. Combine the cranberries, raisins, nuts, and orange rind in a mixing bowl. Combine the beaten egg, orange juice, and oil in a mixing bowl. Stir until everything is well combined. Scrape into a 9 x 5 x 3-inch loaf pan that has been oiled.
2. Preheat the oven to 350 degrees F and bake for one hour, or until a toothpick inserted in the center comes out clean. Allow ten minutes to cool in the pan. Remove the cake from the pan and place it on a wire rack to cool fully.

CRANBERRY ORANGE BREAKFAST BREAD

Preparation: 5 Minutes

Cook: 3 hrs

Servings: 12

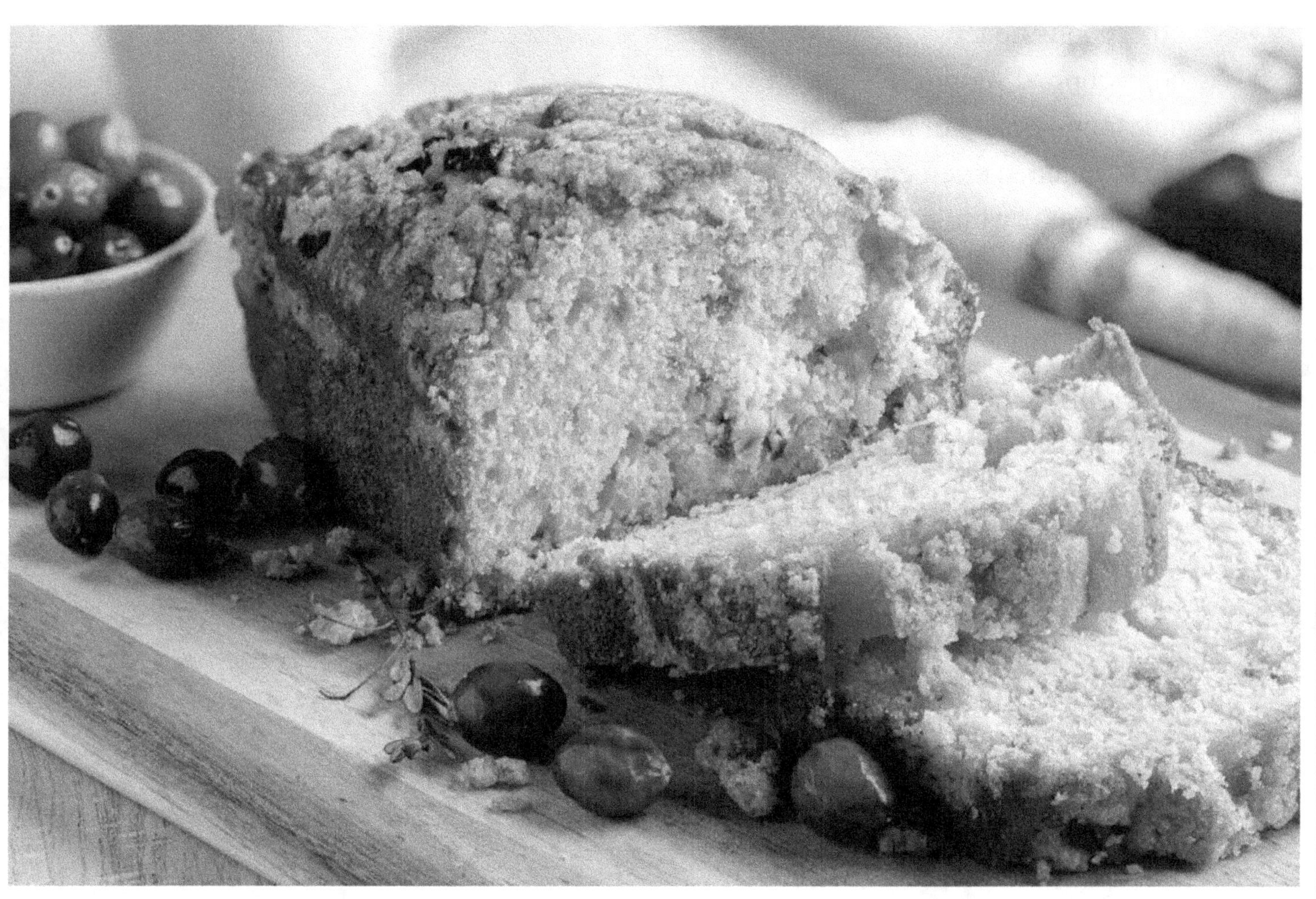

Breakfast, lunch, or just a snack, this rich and hearty fruit bread is perfect. For Thanksgiving, my in-laws devoured it

Nutrition

Calorics: 224 | Protein: 5.2g | Fat: 5.1g | Cholesterol: 0.1mg | Sodium: 198.6mg

Carbohydrates: 39.7g

Ingredients

- ½ teaspoon ground cinnamon
- ½ teaspoon ground allspice
- 1 teaspoon salt
- 1 ⅛ cups orange juice
- 1 package active dry yeast
- 2 tablespoons vegetable oil
- 2 tablespoons honey
- ⅓ cup chopped walnuts 3 cups bread flour
- 1 tablespoon grated orange zest
- 1 cup sweetened dried cranberries
- 1 tablespoon dry milk powder

Instructions

1. Place the ingredients in the bread machine pan in the manufacturer's recommended order.
2. Choose a cycle and press the Start button. If your machine has a Fruit setting, add the cranberries and nuts when the machine beeps, which should be roughly five minutes before the kneading cycle ends.

SWEET POTATO CRANBERRY SAUCE BREAD

Preparation: 20 Minutes

Cook: 45 Minutes

Servings: 12

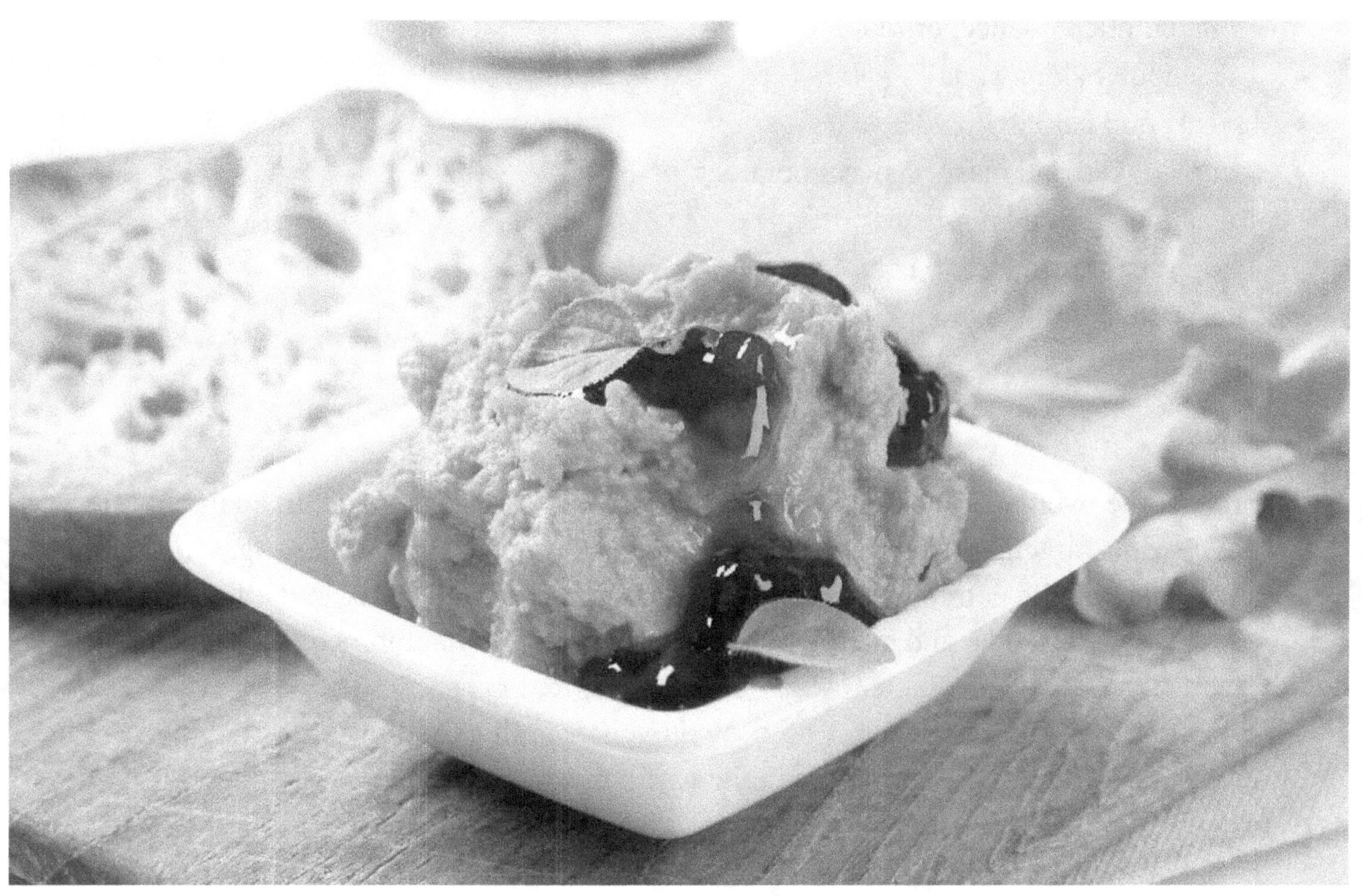

This recipe makes use of two leftovers from the holidays. It has a deliciously festive flavor and is really moist! This is something we made up based on another recipe. You can follow suit. we adore the flavor combination of nutmeg and allspice screams "Christmas" to me.

Nutrition

Calories: 374 | Protein: 5.3g | Cholesterol: 46.5mg | Sodium: 153.1mg

Carbohydrates: 65.6g | Fat: 10.8g

Ingredients

- 3 eggs
- 3 cups all-purpose flour
- ¾ cup white sugar
- 1 teaspoon ground allspice
- ½ cup vegetable oil
- ½ cup brown sugar
- 1 cup cranberry sauce, or more to taste
- 1 teaspoon baking soda
- ½ teaspoon baking powder
- 1 cup cooked and mashed sweet potatoes
- 1 teaspoon ground nutmeg
- 1 cup raisins, or more to taste
- 1 teaspoon vanilla extract

Instructions

1. Preheat the oven to 350 degrees Fahrenheit Grease 4 mini loaf pans. In a large mixing bowl, whisk together the cranberry sauce, sweet potatoes, eggs, white sugar, oil, brown sugar, and vanilla extract with an electric mixer until smooth. Mix in the flour, nutmeg, allspice, baking soda, and baking powder until thoroughly combined. Incorporate the raisins to distribute the batter evenly between the loaf pans.
2. Bake for forty-five minutes in a preheated oven or until a toothpick inserted in the center comes out clean. Cool thoroughly in the loaf pans on a wire rack.

CRANBERRY SCONES

Preparation: 15 Minutes

Cook: 20 Minutes

Servings: 10

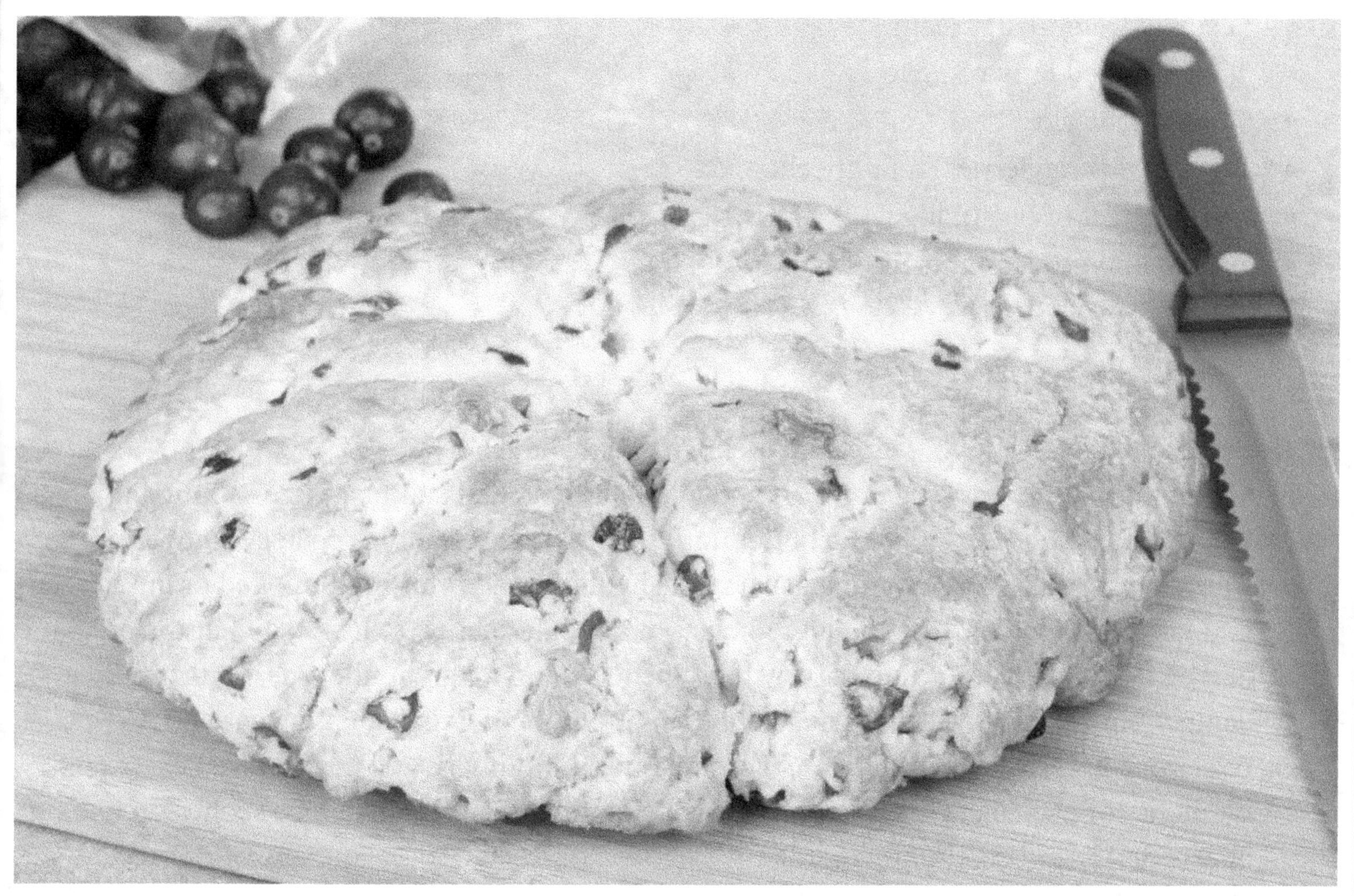

A simple scone recipe made with traditional Christmas ingredients, which is perfect for Christmas morning! Warm, with butter and tea on the side.

Nutrition

Calories: 211 | Protein: 4g | Cholesterol: 31.3mg | Sodium: 173.6mg

Carbohydrates: 28.6g | Fat 9.4g

Ingredients

- 1 egg
- ⅓ cup white sugar
- ½ cup chopped walnuts
- 1 tablespoon baking powder
- 2 cups all-purpose flour
- ¼ cup butter, chilled and diced
- ¾ cup half-and-half cream
- ¼ cup packed brown sugar
- ¼ teaspoon salt
- 1 cup fresh cranberries, roughly chopped
- 1 grated zest of one orange
- ¼ teaspoon ground nutmeg

Instructions

1. Preheat the oven to 375 degrees Fahrenheit (190 degrees C).
2. Combine flour, brown sugar, baking powder, nutmeg, and salt in a large mixing bowl. Using a pastry cutter, cut in the butter until the mixture resembles coarse crumbs.
3. Toss cranberries with sugar in a separate dish; add to the flour mixture, and orange peel and nuts. Lightly combine the ingredients. In a separate bowl, whisk together the cream and egg; gradually pour into the dry ingredients, scraping down the sides with a rubber scraper until a dough forms. Knead the dough four or five times, taking care not to overwork it. Divide dough in half. Turn out onto a floured work surface. Make a 6-inch circle out of each half. Each circular must be cut into six wedges. Place scones on baking sheets that have been lightly oiled.
4. Bake for twenty minutes in a preheated oven until golden brown.

CITRUS CRANBERRY ZUCCHINI BREAD

Preparation: 15 Minutes

Cook: 1 hr 10 Minutes

Servings: 10

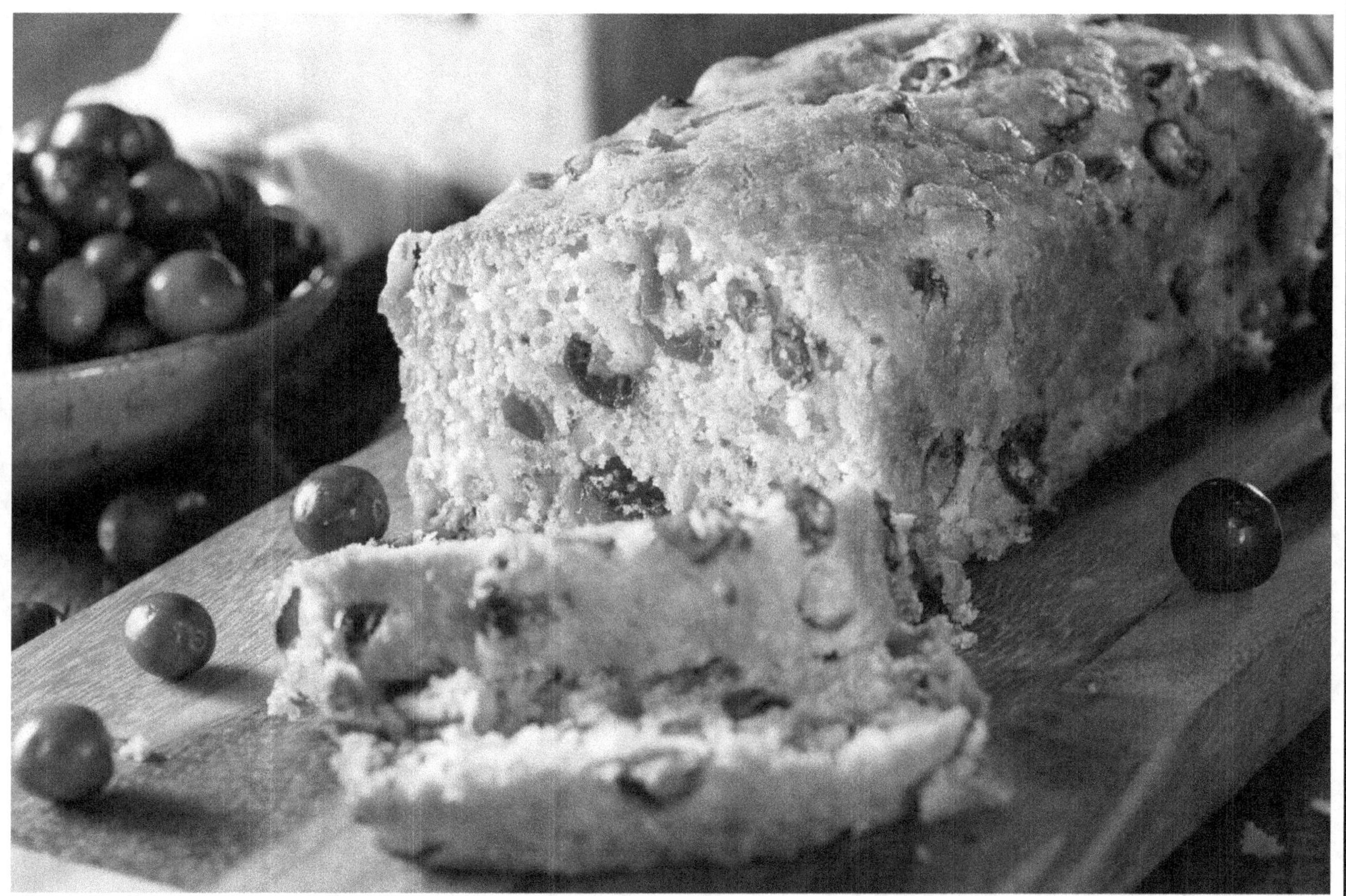

Zucchini bread with a flavor of lemon and orange, accentuated by dried cranberries, is a delectable take on a summer favorite.

Nutrition

Calories: 270 | Protein: 4.3g | Cholesterol: 30.8mg | Sodium: 390.2mg

Carbohydrates: 43.9g | Fat: 9.2g

Ingredients

- 3 eggs
- 2 cups shredded zucchini
- 1 cup dried cranberries
- 2 cups white sugar
- 3 cups all-purpose flour
- ¼ teaspoon baking powder
- 1 cup vegetable oil
- 1 teaspoon baking soda
- 2 teaspoons ground cinnamon
- 1 teaspoon ground cloves
- 1 teaspoon ground nutmeg
- 1 teaspoon salt
- 1 teaspoon lemon extract
- 1 orange, zested
- 1 pinch ground ginger

Instructions

1. Preheat the oven to 325°F. Grease two 8x4-inch loaf pans.
2. In a small mixing bowl, combine flour, baking soda, and baking powder. In a large mixing dish, whisk the eggs with the sugar until thoroughly combined, then add the oil. In a mixing bowl, combine zucchini, cranberries, orange zest, and lemon extract. Mix the cinnamon, cloves, nutmeg, salt, and ginger in a bowl.
3. Bake in the preheated oven for fifty to sixty minutes, or until a toothpick inserted in the center comes out clean. Cool for ten minutes in the pans before removing to a wire rack to cool fully.

CRANBERRY BANANA OAT BREAD

Preparation: 15 Minutes

Cook: 50 Minutes

Servings: 24

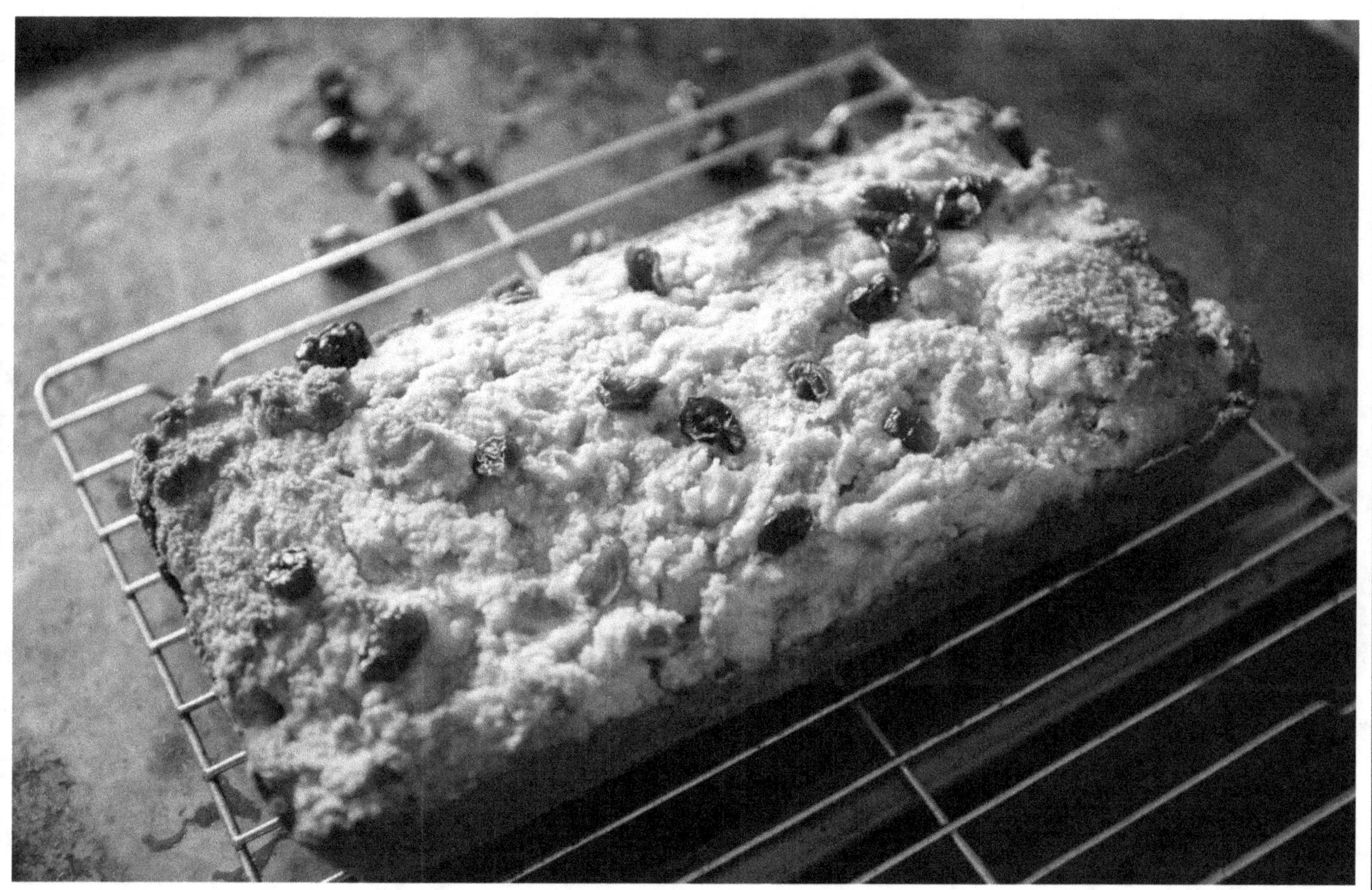

Banana bread with a twist. The cranberries provide a sweet and tangy flavor to the bread that truly brings it to life. It's a terrific addition to brunch because it's incredibly moist and tasty! Try brushing the top of the baked loaf with melted butter and a pastry brush if you prefer a more buttery flavor.

Nutrition

Calories: 230 | Protein: 2.6g | Cholesterol: 23.3mg | Sodium: 164.8mg

Carbohydrates: 33.5g | Fat: 9.9g

Ingredients

- 2 large eggs
- 1 ¼ cups all-purpose flour
- 1 ¼ cups mashed ripe bananas
- 2 tablespoons sour cream
- 1 cup quick-cooking oats
- ¾ cup dried cranberries
- ½ teaspoon lemon juice
- ½ cup white sugar
- ⅓ cup melted butter
- 1 tablespoon baking powder
- ½ teaspoon salt

Instructions

1. Preheat oven to 350 degrees Fahrenheit. Grease a 2 1/2 x 8 1/2-inch loaf pan with butter. In a mixing bowl, combine the flour, oats, baking powder, and salt; set aside.
2. In a mixing dish, whisk the eggs until smooth. Combine the bananas, sour cream, and melted butter in a mixing bowl. Mix in the sugar, cranberries, and lemon juice until well combined. Fold into the oat mixture until there are no dry lumps. Pour into the loaf pan that has been prepared.
3. Bake in the preheated oven until a toothpick inserted into the center comes out clean, forty to fifty minutes Cool for ten minutes in the pans before removing to a wire rack to cool fully.

CRANBERRY OAT BREAD

Preparation: 15 Minutes

Cook: 45 Minutes

Servings: 10

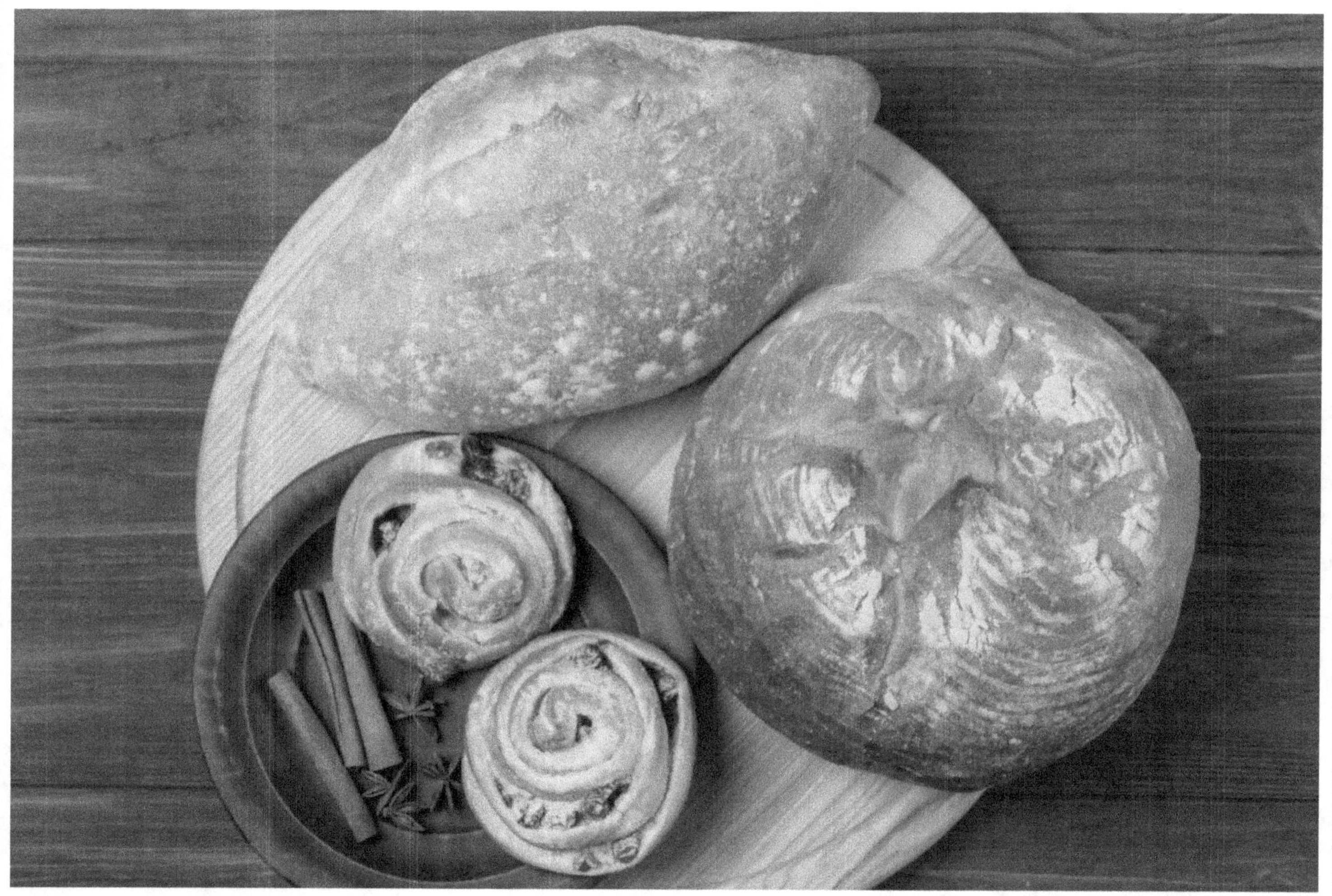

This is a delicious, moist bread that you can make in a bread machine. This recipe makes a one-and-a-half-pound loaf of bread.

Nutrition

Calories: 254 | Protein: 4.4g | Cholesterol: 54.7mg | Sodium: 322.7mg

Carbohydrates: 41.9g | Fat: 8.5g

Ingredients

- 1 cup water
- 2 tablespoons honey
- ⅓ cup rolled oats
- 2 ½ cups bread flour
- ¾ teaspoon salt
- ½ teaspoon ground cinnamon
- 1 tablespoon butter, softened
- 1 ¾ teaspoon active dry yeast
- package dried cranberries

Instructions

1. In the bread machine's pan, add water, butter, honey, salt, cinnamon, oats, bread flour, yeast, and dried cranberries in the sequence advised by the manufacturer.
2. Select the Basic Bread cycle and press the Start button.

CRANBERRY APPLE BREAD

Preparation: 30 Minutes

Cook: 45 Minutes

Servings: 12

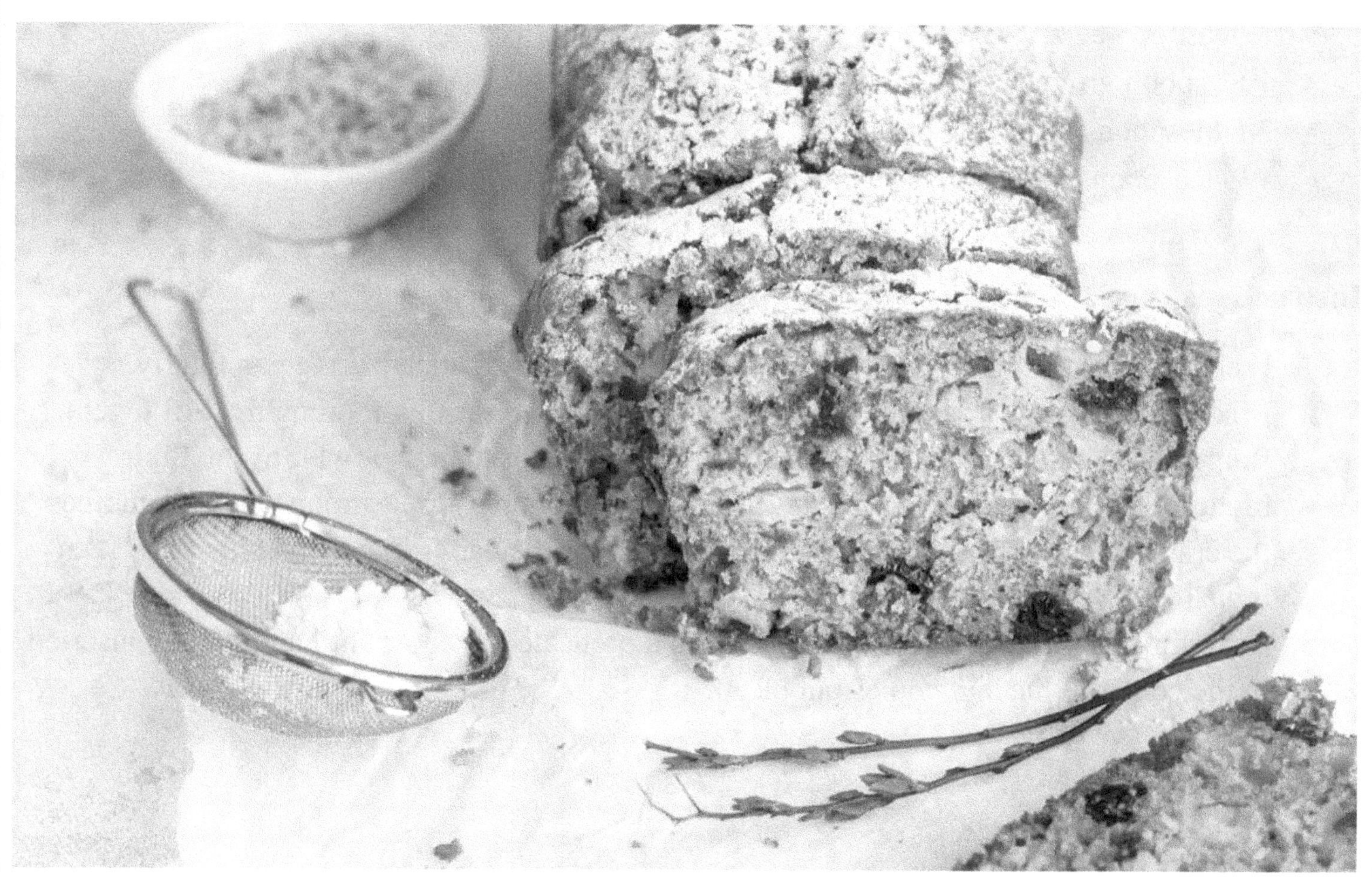

In our family, this bread is a holiday classic. It's a festive breakfast bread that's perfect for Thanksgiving and Christmas mornings. We prefer to make my bread batter ahead of time and then thaw it the night before serving. Simply drop it in the oven first thing in the morning for fresh breakfast bread. Enjoy

Nutrition

Calories: 179 | Protein: 3g | Cholesterol: 15.5mg | Sodium: 104mg

Carbohydrates: 29.3g | Fat: 6.1g

Ingredients

- 1 egg
- 1 ½ cups all-purpose flour
- 1 cup fresh or frozen cranberries
- 2 cups peeled, cored, and chopped apple
- ½ cup chopped walnuts
- ¾ cup white sugar
- ½ teaspoon baking soda
- 1 teaspoon ground cinnamon
- 2 tablespoons vegetable oil
- 1 ½ teaspoons baking powder

Instructions

1. Preheat the oven to 350 degrees Fahrenheit. Grease a 9x5-inch baking pan lightly.
2. Mix the apples, sugar, and oil in a mixing bowl. Mix in the egg thoroughly. Sift together flour, baking powder, baking soda, and cinnamon in a separate bowl. Stir the flour mixture into the wet ingredients until the dry components are just moistened. Combine the cranberries and walnuts in a mixing bowl. Pour the batter into the pan that has been prepared.
3. Bake for thirty-five to forty-five minutes in a preheated oven or until a toothpick inserted in the center of the loaf comes out clean.

CHALLAH RECIPE

Preparation: 30 Minutes

Cook:40 Minutes

Servings: 30

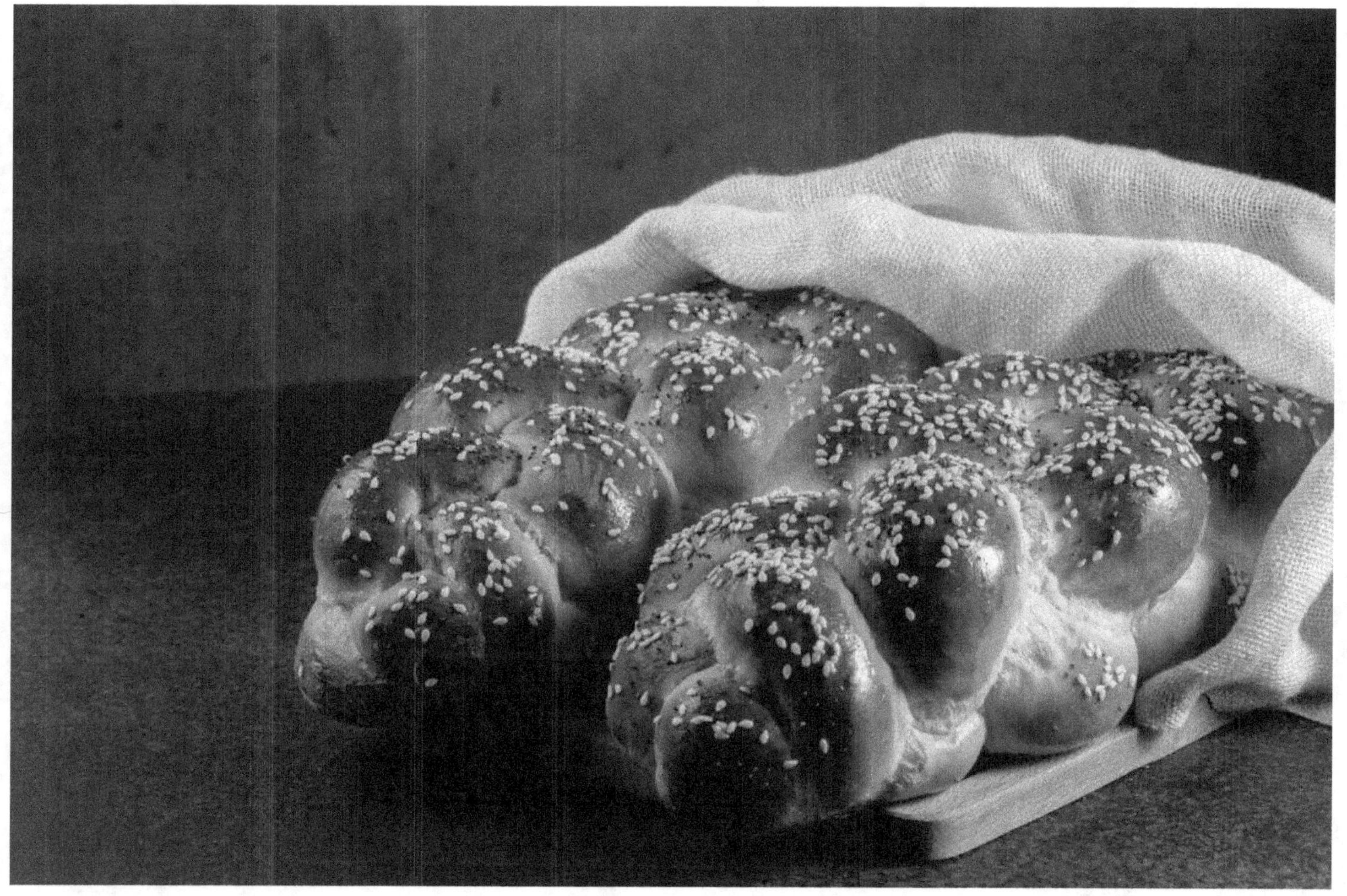

For the Jewish Sabbath, traditional egg bread is made. One cup of raisins or golden raisins can be added to the dough right before shaping and then shaped into round loaves.

Nutrition

Calories: 165 | Protein: 4.3g | Cholesterol: 18.6mg | Sodium: 241.3mg

Carbohydrates: 30.3g | Fat: 2.8g

Ingredients

- 3 eggs
- 1 tablespoon salt
- ½ cup honey
- 8 cups unbleached all-purpose flour
- 2 ½ cups warm water
- 1 tablespoon active dry yeast
- 4 tablespoons vegetable oil
- 1 tablespoon poppy seeds (Optional)

Instructions

1. Sprinkle yeast over barely warm water in a large mixing bowl. Honey, oil, 2 eggs, and salt are combined in a mixing bowl. As the dough thickens, add the flour one cup at a time, beating after each addition and progressing to kneading with hands. Knead until the dough is smooth, elastic, and not sticky, adding flour as required. Allow dough to rise for one and half hours or until it has doubled in size.
2. Turn out the dough onto a floured surface when it has risen. Divide the dough in half and knead each half for about five minutes, adding flour as required to keep it from sticking.
3. Divide each piece into thirds and wrap it into a long snake with a diameter of about 1 1/2 inches. Braid from the middle, tightly pinching the ends of the three snakes together. Curling the braid into a round, and squeezing the ends together. Leave as it is, or make into a round braided loaf by bringing the ends together.
4. Place the final braid or circle on each of two baking trays that have been greased. Cover with a towel and set aside for one hour to rise.
5. Preheat the oven to 375 degrees Fahrenheit
6. Brush a good amount of the remaining egg over each braid. If desired, top with poppy seeds.
7. Preheat oven to 375 degrees F and bake for forty minutes. When you hit the bottom of the bread, it should make a beautiful hollow sound before slicing, cool for at least one hour on a rack.

BRIOCHE

Preparation: 40 Minutes

Cook: 30 Minutes

Servings: 16

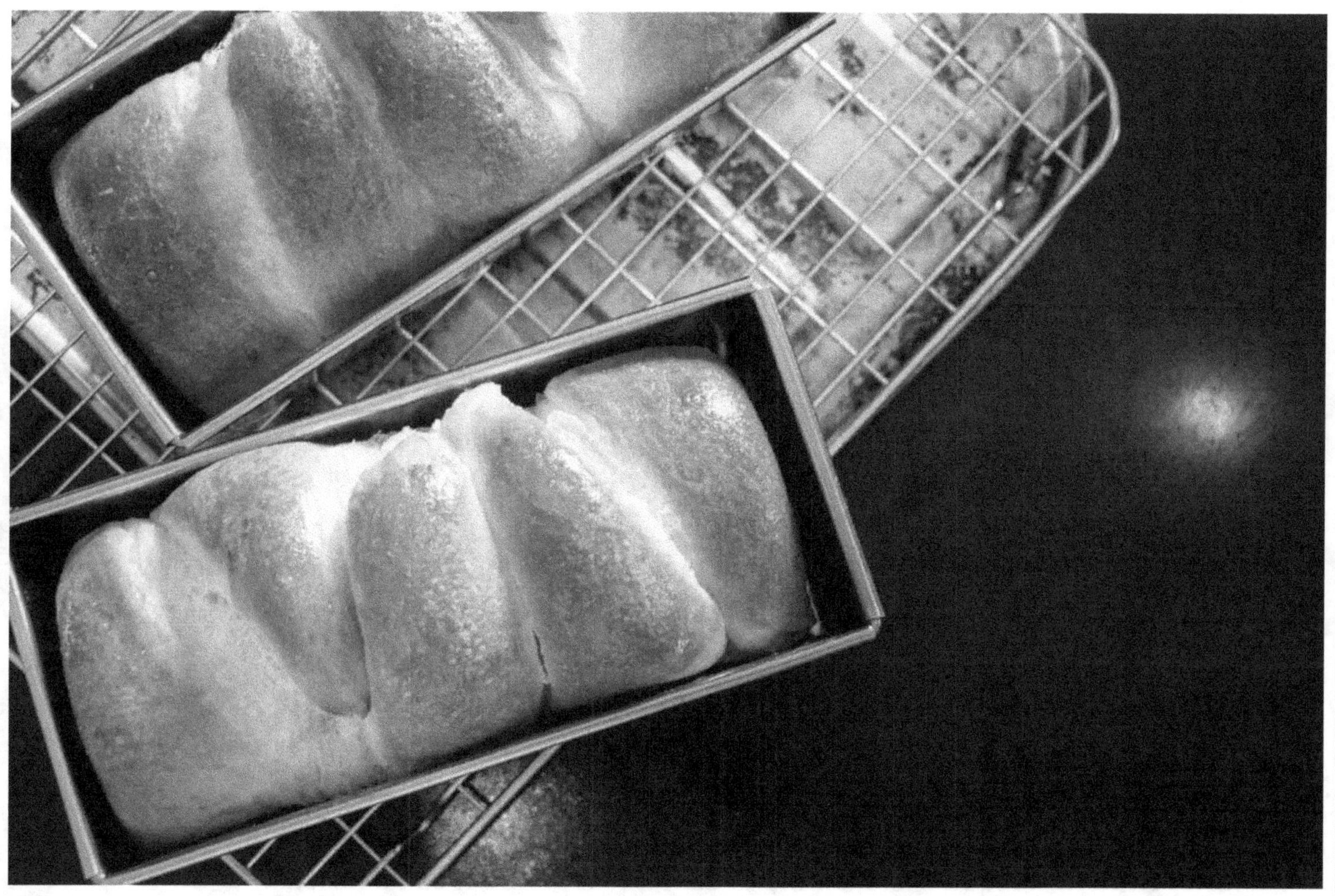

With tea or coffee, a fresh brioche can be served with jelly or other preserves or with pate or hors d'oeuvres. The small ones' caps can simply be taken away, revealing a sweet or savory inside. Brioche dough can also be used to wrap other things like meat for boeuf en croûte, salmon for a koulibiaca, or spicy garlic sausage.

Nutrition

Calories: 228 | Protein: 5g | Cholesterol: 89.8mg | Sodium: 246.1mg

Carbohydrates: 22.1g | Fat: 13.3g

Ingredients

- 4 eggs
- 1 egg yolk
- 1 teaspoon cold water
- 1 tablespoon white sugar
- 1 tablespoon active dry yeast
- ⅓ cup warm water
- 3 ½ cups all-purpose flour
- 1 cup butter, softened
- 1 teaspoon salt

Instructions

1. Dissolve yeast in warm water in a small bowl. Allow ten minutes for the mixture to become creamy.
2. Combine the flour, sugar, and salt in a large mixing bowl. In the center of the bowl, make a well and add the eggs and yeast mixture. After the dough has pulled together, roll it out onto a lightly floured surface and knead for about eight minutes, or until smooth and supple.
3. Spread one-third of the butter on the dough and flatten it. Knead this thoroughly. To incorporate the remaining butter, repeat the process twice more. Allow for a few minutes of resting time between butter additions. This procedure could take up to twenty minutes. Lightly grease a large mixing bowl, then set the dough in it and turn to coat it in oil. Cover with plastic wrap and set aside in a warm place to rise for one hour or until doubled in volume.
4. Deflate the dough, wrap it with plastic wrap, and place it in the refrigerator for six hours or overnight. It requires some time to cool down before it can be used.
5. On a lightly floured surface, roll out the dough. Cover with oiled plastic wrap and let rise for about 60 minutes, or until doubled in volume. Divide the dough into two equal portions, shape it into loaves, and bake in the prepared pans.
6. Preheat the oven to 400 degrees Fahrenheit. To make rolls, lightly butter two 9x5-inch loaf pans. To prepare a glaze, whisk together the egg yolk and 1 teaspoon of water.
7. Brush the egg wash on the loaves or rolls. Bake till golden brown in a preheated oven. After twenty-five minutes, check the loaves for doneness, and after ten minutes, roll them out. Allow ten minutes for the loaves to cool in the pans before transferring them to wire racks to cool entirely.

CHEESE BABKA

Preparation: 1 hour

Cook: 40 Minutes

Servings: 12

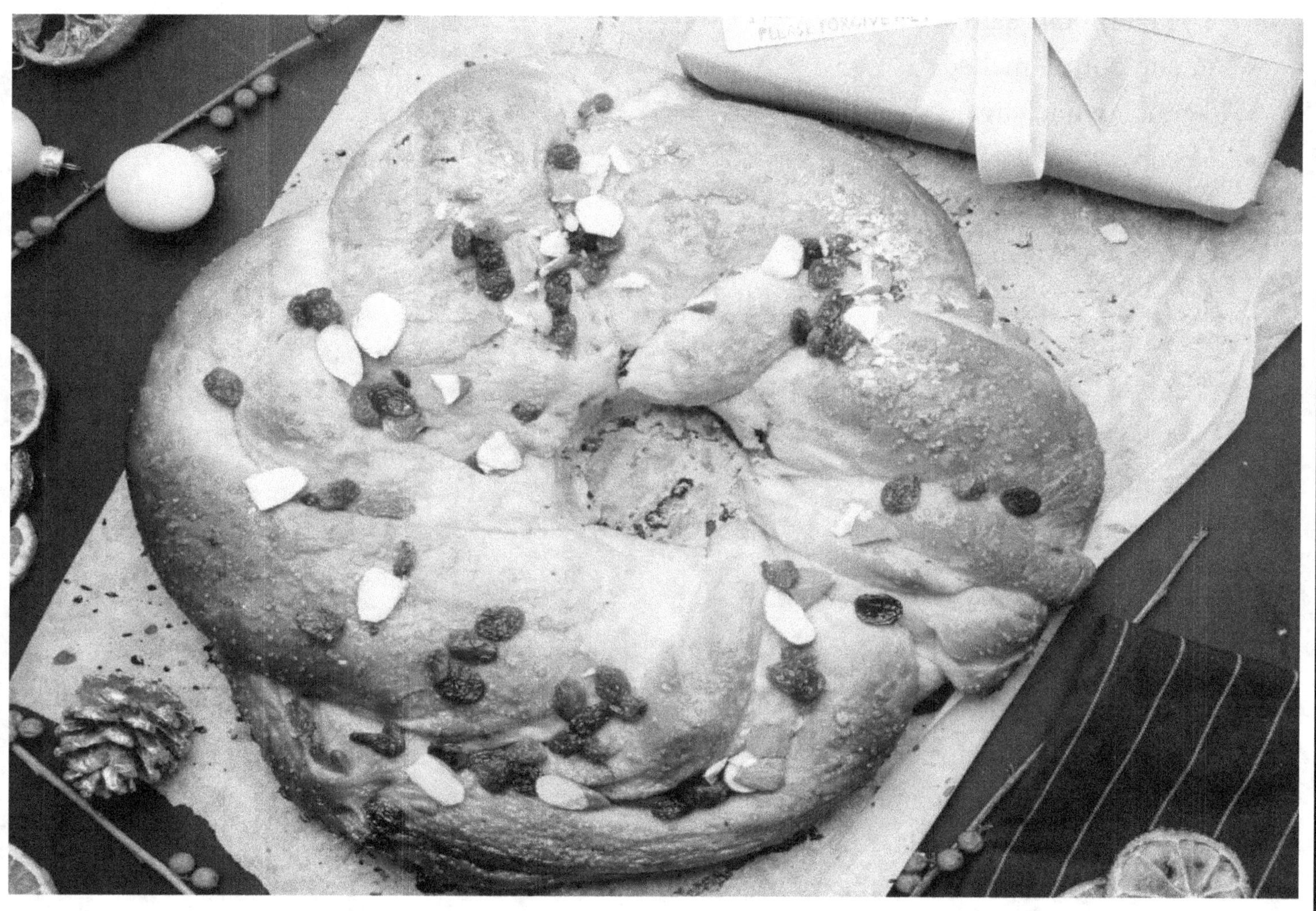

Every Easter, Polish cheese babka is offered.

Nutrition

Calories: 513 | Protein: 19.1g | Carbohydrates: 44g | Fat: 28.2g

Cholesterol: 133.9mg | Sodium: 768.6mg

Ingredients

<u>Dough</u>

- 3 eggs
- 4 cups all-purpose flour, divided
- 1 package active dry yeast
- ¼ cup white sugar
- 1 ½ teaspoons salt
- ½ cup butter, melted
- 1 pinch white sugar
- ¼ cup warm water
- 2 teaspoons vanilla extract
- ¾ cup lukewarm milk

<u>Filling</u>

- 1 egg
- 1 teaspoon vanilla extract
- 1 ½ cups farmers cheese
- ½ teaspoon dried lemon peel ⅓ cup white sugar
- 2 tablespoons butter, melted 1 ½ tablespoons sour cream

Instructions

1. Over the warm water, sprinkle the yeast and a pinch of sugar and stir to dissolve. Allow ten minutes for the foam to form. In a mixing dish, combine 1/2 cup butter, 1/4 cup sugar, salt, 2 teaspoons vanilla, milk, and 3 eggs, along with 1 cup flour. one minute after adding the yeast mixture, beat for another minute.
2. Add the remaining flour in a slow, steady stream to make a soft dough. Knead the dough until smooth and elastic on a lightly floured surface, adding small quantities of flour as needed to keep it from sticking. Form a circle out of the dough and lay it in an oiled bowl, turning to coat. Allow the dough to rise at room temperature until it has doubled in size, about one and half hours.
3. In a mixing dish, combine the farmers' cheese, 1/3 cup sugar, sour cream, 1 egg, 1 teaspoon vanilla extract, and dried lemon peel. Remove the filling from the pan and set it aside. A 10-inch fluted tube pan should be lightly oiled. Pat the dough into a 10-inch by 12-inch rectangle on a lightly floured surface. Take 2 tablespoons of melted butter to brush on the dough. Evenly spread the cheese filling over the dough.

4. Starting from the long end, roll the dough up like a jelly roll; twist the dough six to eight times to form a rope. Pinch the seams and ends shut, then place the dough rope in the buttered pan. Cover loosely and set aside for one hour to rise.
5. Preheat the oven to 350 degrees Fahrenheit.
6. Bake the babka for forty to forty-five minutes, or until golden brown. Remove the babka from the oven and set it aside for five minutes before inverting it onto a wire rack and removing the pan. Allow at least two hours for the babka to cool before slicing.'

NUMBER ONE EGG BREAD

Preparation: 20 Minutes

Cook: 40 Minutes

Servings: 18

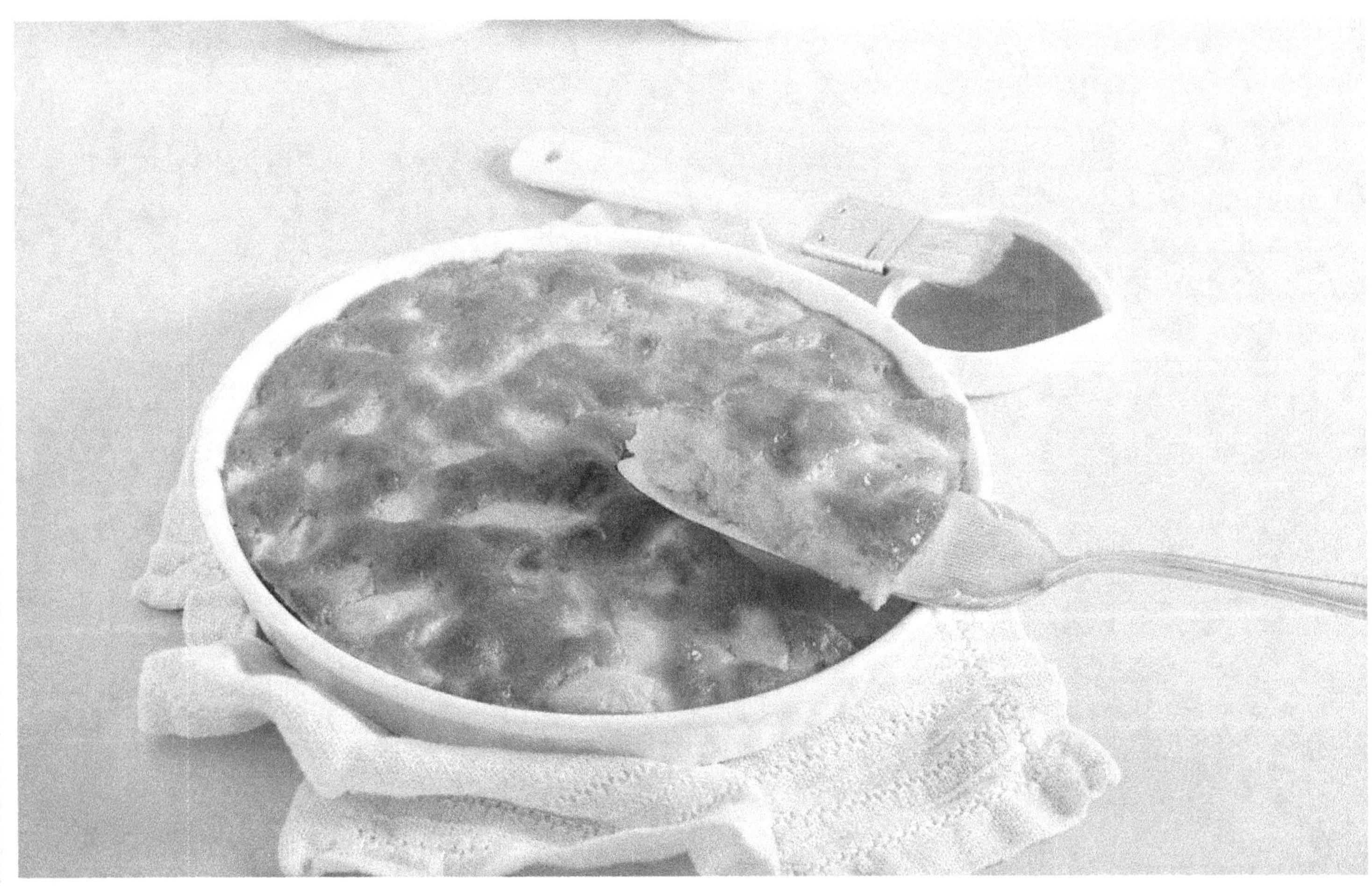

All other egg bread pale in comparison. In Hawaii, we learned the dish from two older ladies. This recipe yields the finest bread pudding and french toast you've ever had. Cut it into bits and dip it in the fondue-style sauce.

Nutrition

Calories: 214 | Protein: 5.8g | Cholesterol: 109.6mg | Sodium: 148.4mg

Carbohydrates: 27.2g | Fat: 9g

Ingredients

- 1 egg
- 6 egg yolks
- 4 ½ cups all-purpose flour
- 3 eggs, room temperature
- ½ cup vegetable oil
- 2 packages of active dry yeast
- ⅔ cup warm water
- ¼ cup white sugar
- 1 teaspoon salt
- 1 pinch salt

Instructions

1. Dissolve yeast in water in a large mixing dish. Combine the yolks, 3 eggs, oil, sugar, and salt in a mixing bowl. To make a sticky dough, add roughly 3-1/2 cups of flour. Turn out the dough onto a floured surface. Knead for seven minutes with the remaining flour until smooth and elastic. Place the dough in a well-oiled bowl and turn to coat the entire surface. Using a moist cloth, cover the dish. Area in a warm place for about 1-1/2 hours, or until doubled in size.
2. Divide the dough into three pieces after punching it down. Make a rope out of each piece that is about 12 inches long. Braid the three strands together and secure the ends with a rubber band. Place the bread on a cookie sheet that has been buttered. Brush the remaining 1 egg on the bread with a pinch of salt. Allow the bread to rise for forty-five minutes or until it has doubled in size.
3. Preheat the oven to 375°F. Brush the bread with the egg wash once more.
4. Preheat oven to 400°F and bake for forty minutes, or until golden brown. Allow it to cool on a wire rack.

BREAD MACHINE CHALLAH RECIPE

Preparation: 30 Minutes

Cook: 25 Minutes

Servings: 20

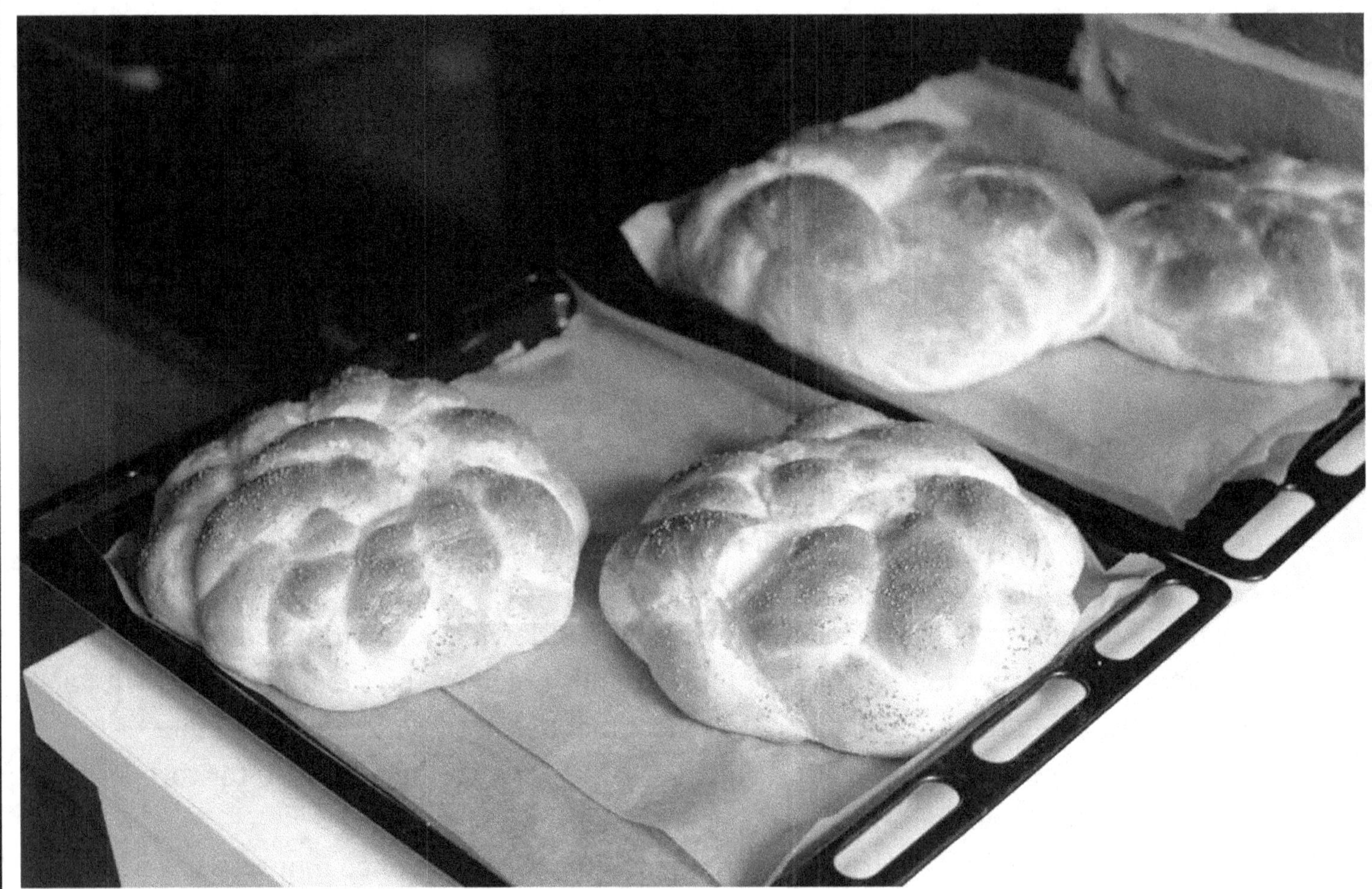

Exceptionally tasty. We have a two-pound bread machine that we use to make the dough for the Challah. It keeps well in the freezer.

Nutrition

Calories: 182 | Protein: 4.4g | Cholesterol: 27.9mg | Sodium: 302mg

Carbohydrates: 26g | Fat: 6.7g

Ingredients

- 1 egg, beaten
- 1 tablespoon water
- 2 large eggs, room temperature
- 2 ¼ teaspoons bread machine yeast
- 4 cups bread flour
- 1 cup warm water
- ½ cup white sugar
- 1 tablespoon honey
- ½ cup vegetable oil
- 2 ½ teaspoons salt

Instructions

1. Fill the bread machine pan with warm water, sugar, honey, vegetable oil, salt, 2 eggs, flour, and yeast in the sequence indicated by the manufacturer. Select the Dough cycle and push the Start button.
2. Take the dough out of the machine and set it on a lightly floured surface, punch it down, and let it rest for five minutes.
3. Make a half-dozen cuts in the dough. Then divide into three equal halves, roll into 12- to 14-inch ropes, and braid into a loaf. Carry out the same procedure with the remaining half. Environment the loaves on a greased cookie sheet, spritz with water, cover loosely with plastic wrap and let rise in a warm, draft-free place for one and half hours, or until doubled in size.
4. Preheat the oven to 350 degrees Fahrenheit . 1 egg and 1 tablespoon water, whisked together in a small bowl.
5. Brush the egg mixture on the risen bread. Cook for twenty to twenty-five minutes in a preheated oven. Cover with foil if it starts to brown too quickly.

CHALLAH BREAD NEW RECIPE 2

Preparation: 25 Minutes

Cook: 30 Minutes

Servings: 10

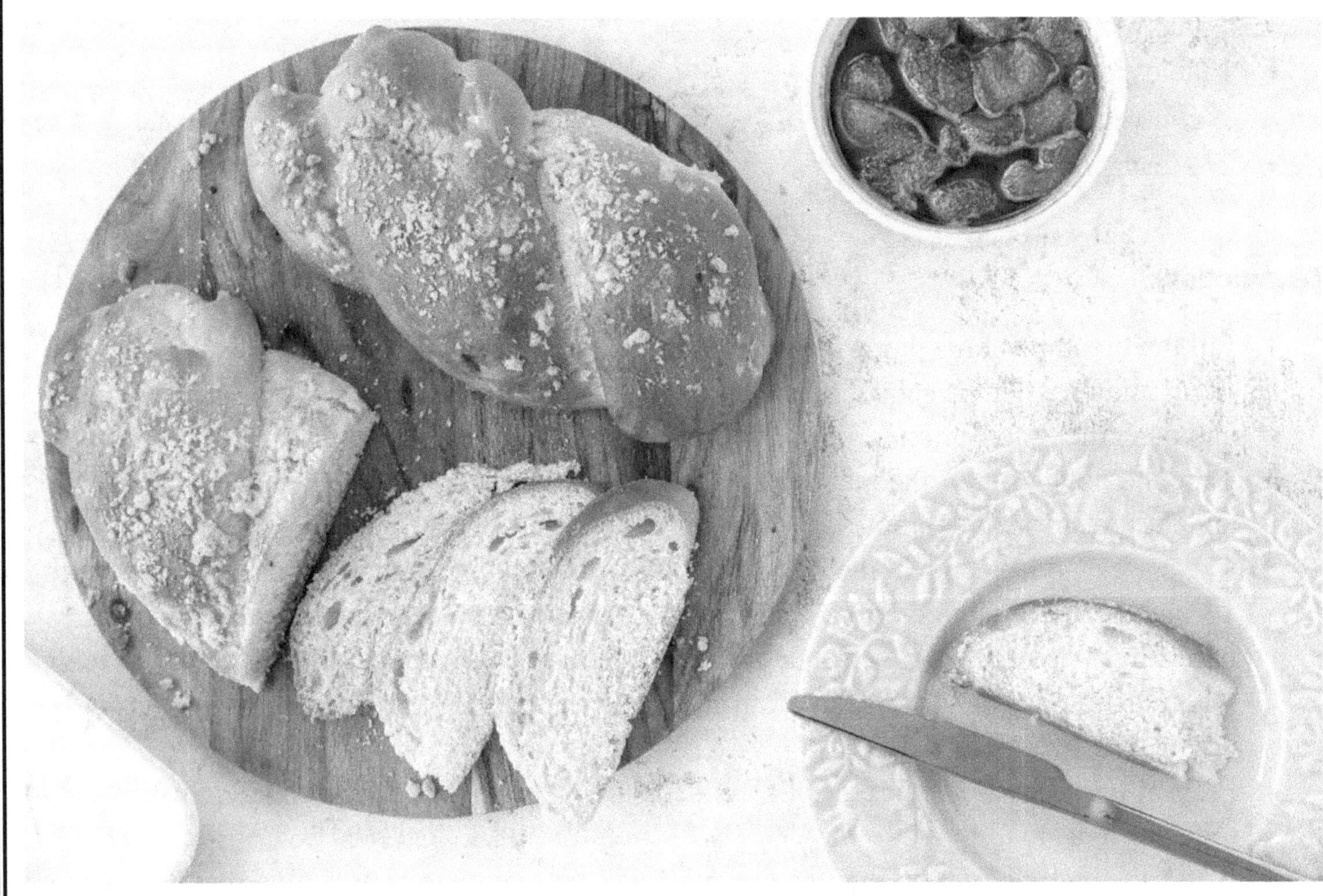

This Challah Bread recipe yields two of the most beautiful braided loaves you'll ever eat! Enjoy one loaf while it's still warm from the oven, and keep the other for French toast a few days later!

Nutrition

Calories: 211 | Protein: 7g | Cholesterol: 79.3mg | Sodium: 264.6mg

Carbohydrates: 37.3g | Fat: 3.5g

Ingredients

- 3 beaten eggs
- 1 cup warm water
- 2 tablespoons honey 3 ½ cups all-purpose flour, plus more for kneading
- package active dry yeast
- 1 tablespoon melted butter (optional)
- 1 teaspoon salt

Instructions

1. Stir the yeast into the water in a large mixing bowl and set aside for ten minutes, or until a creamy layer develops on top. Stir in the honey and salt until they are completely dissolved, then add the beaten eggs. Add a cup of flour at a time until the dough is sticky. Dust the dough with flour and knead for five minutes, or until smooth and elastic.
2. Place the dough in an oiled dish and shape it into a tight spherical shape. Turn the dough over in the bowl several times to oil the surface, cover with a wet cloth, and let rise in a warm place until doubled in size, forty-five minutes to one hour. Punch down the dough and divide it into three pieces of equal size. Roll the little dough pieces into ropes about the thickness of your thumb and about 12 inches long on a floured surface. The center of the rope should be thicker than the ends, and the ends should be thinner. Braid three ropes at the top by pinching them together. Move the strand to the left over the center strand, starting with the strand to the right.
3. Move the strand that is furthest to the left over the new middle strand. Continue braiding until the loaf is braided, alternating sides each time, and squeeze the ends together and fold them underneath for a clean look. Brush the top of the braided loaf with beaten egg yolk and place it on a baking sheet lined with parchment paper.
4. Preheat the oven to 350 degrees Fahrenheit.
5. Bake the Challah in the preheated oven for thirty to thirty-five minutes, or until the top is a rich golden color and the loaf sounds hollow when tapped with a spoon. Before slicing, cool on a wire rack.

KHOBZ EL DAR, ALGERIAN SEMOLINA BREAD

Preparation: 30 Minutes

Cook: 20 Minutes

Servings: 8

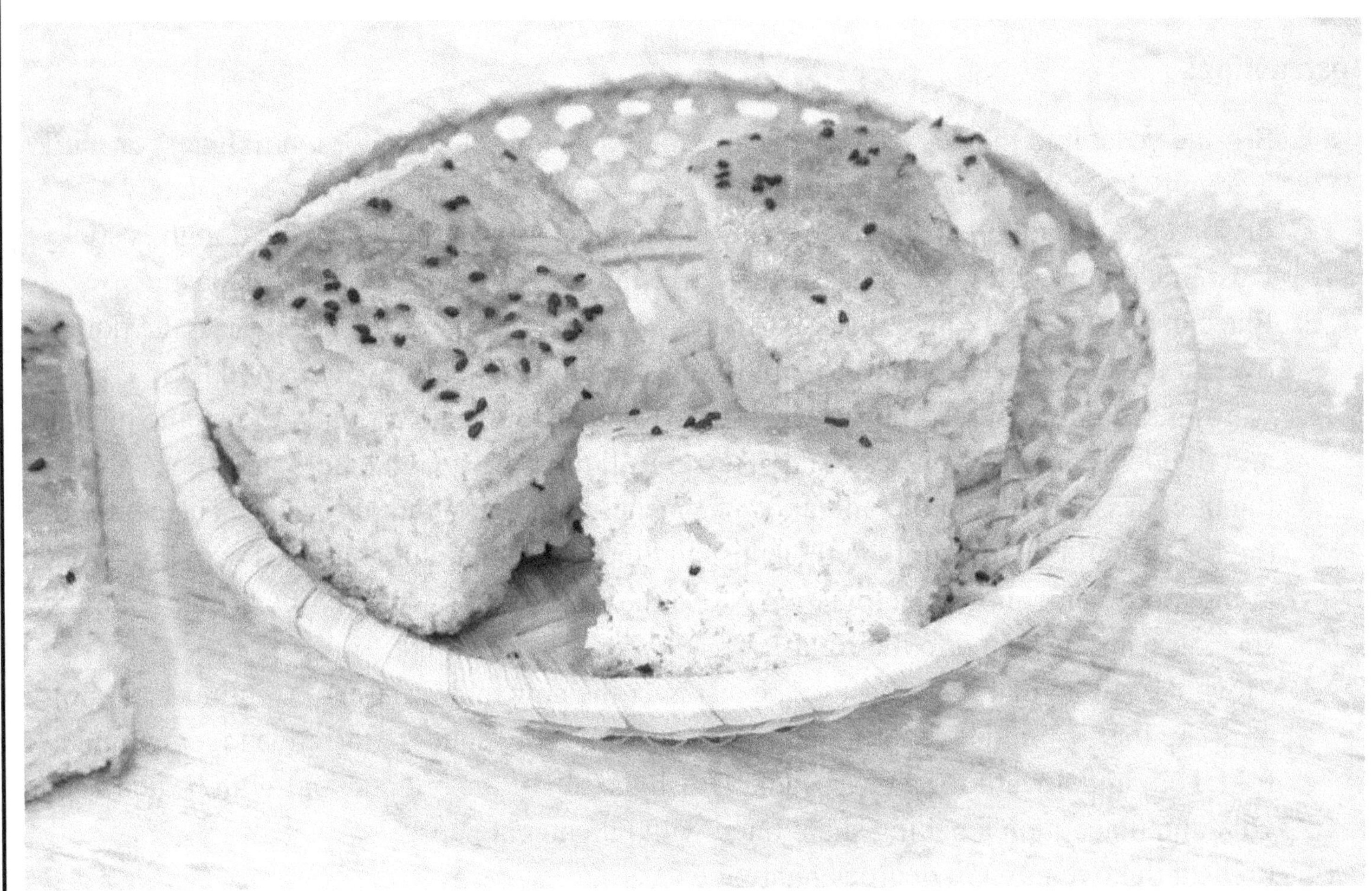

If you've never had Algerian bread before, you should certainly try this quick and easy recipe. It's called Khobz el Dar because it doesn't require any kneading, sophisticated methods, or anything more than basic ingredients. The outcome is a brioche-like bread that is extremely soft and somewhat sweet. Exceptionally tasty.

Nutrition

Calories: 293 | Protein: 8.3g | Carbohydrates: 40.2g | Cholesterol: 48.9mg

Sodium: 249.6mg | Fat: 10.8g

Ingredients

- 1 egg
- 1 egg, separated
- 2 ¾ cups all-purpose flour
- 1 teaspoon water
- ½ cup semolina flour
- 2 tablespoons all-purpose flour, or more as needed
- 2 tablespoons semolina flour
- ¼ cup vegetable oil
- 1 cup lukewarm milk
- 3 tablespoons sesame seeds, divided
- 1 tablespoon white sugar
- 1 teaspoon active dry yeast
- ¾ teaspoon salt

Instructions

1. In a large mixing bowl, combine 1/2 cup plus 2 tablespoons semolina, 2 tablespoons sesame seeds, sugar, yeast, and salt. Combine the oil, egg, and egg white in a mixing bowl. Slowly pour in warm milk until a liquid dough develops.
2. Cover the bowl with a plate or plastic wrap and set aside at room temperature for about one hour or until bubbly.
3. With a wooden spoon, stir in 2 3/4 cups flour until a sticky dough forms. Cover and set aside for another thirty minutes.
4. Using parchment paper or a baking mat, line a baking sheet.
5. Sprinkle 1 tablespoon flour over the dough and your hands. Mix the dough until it pulls away from the sides of the bowl, adding flour as required, 1 tablespoon at a time.
6. Form into a round loaf and place on the baking sheet that has been prepared. Cover loosely with a cloth. And set aside in a warm location for one hour or until the loaf has doubled in size.
7. Preheat the oven to 400 degrees Fahrenheit.
8. In a bowl, whisk together the egg yolk and water with a fork. And brush over the entire surface of the bread. One tablespoon sesame seeds, sprinkled on top.
9. Cook for twenty to twenty-five minutes in a preheated oven until the bread is golden brown.

POTICA

Preparation: 30 Minutes

Cook: 1 hr

Servings: 30

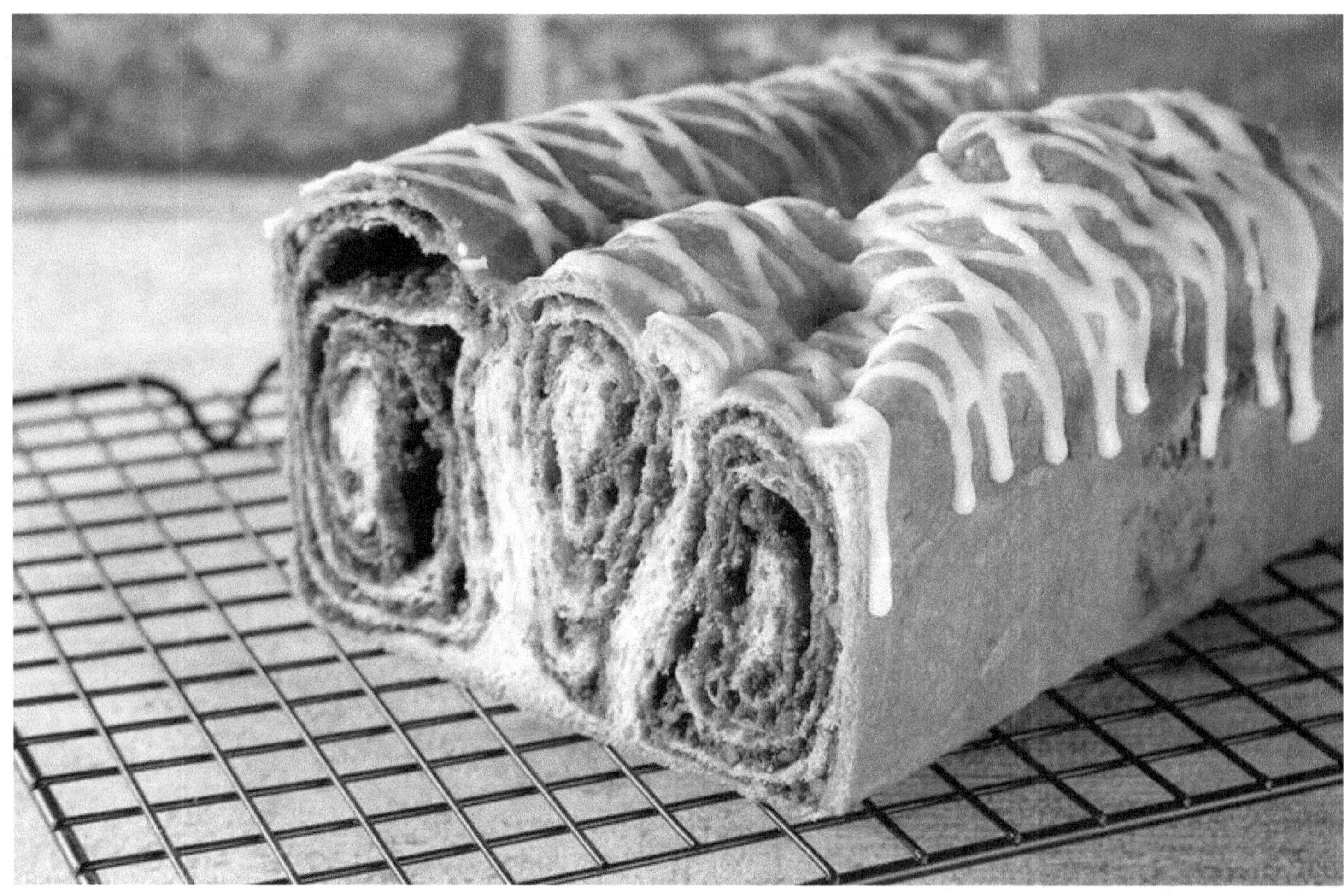

This is a delicious Slovenia bread with a sweet, nutty interior. It's difficult to discover the recipe because of the spelling and pronunciation (paw-tee'-tzah).

Nutrition

Calories: 306 | Protein: 4.5g | Cholesterol: 74.5mg | Sodium: 173.6mg

Carbohydrates: 35.2g | Fat: 17.5g

Ingredients

- 6 egg yolks
- 5 cups all-purpose flour
- 1 ⅓ cups milk
- 1 ½ teaspoons active dry yeast
- ¼ cup white sugar
- 1 tablespoon ground cinnamon
- 1 cup butter, melted
- ¼ cup milk, lukewarm
- 1 ½ cups chopped walnuts
- 1 cup butter, softened
- 1 teaspoon salt
- 1 cup honey
- 1 ½ cups raisins

Instructions

1. Dissolve yeast, 1 teaspoon sugar, and 3 tablespoons flour in warm milk in a small mixing dish. Mix well and let aside for ten minutes, or until creamy.
2. Cream the butter with the remaining sugar in a large mixing bowl. One at a time, add the egg yolks, beating vigorously after each addition. Combine the yeast mixture, remaining milk, 4 cups flour, and salt in a large mixing bowl. Add the remaining flour, 1/2 cup at a time, stirring well after each addition
3. When the dough has come together, turn it out onto a lightly floured surface and knead for about eight minutes, or until smooth and elastic. Lightly grease a large mixing bowl, then set the dough in it and turn to coat it in oil. Cover with a moist towel and set aside in a warm place to rise for one hour or until doubled in volume. Grease one or two cookie sheets lightly. Turn the dough out onto a lightly floured surface to deflate it. Roll out the dough into two equal pieces to a thickness of 1/4 to 1/2 inch. Spread melted butter, honey, raisins, walnuts, and cinnamon on each slice.
4. Pinch the ends of each piece and roll it up like a jelly roll. Place the seam side down on the baking pans that have been prepared. Allow to rise until it has doubled in volume. Preheat the oven to 350 degrees Fahrenheit.
5. Bake for sixty minutes at 350 degrees F golden on top.